The Magic of
MASSAGE
A NEW AND HOLISTIC APPROACH

Revised Edition

The Magic of
MASSAGE
A NEW AND HOLISTIC APPROACH

BY OUIDA WEST, M. TH.

Hastings House
Book Publishers
Mamaroneck, New York

Dedication

This book is dedicated to my parents, and the following people
for the profound influence they have had on my personal and professional life:
Richard Gallen; Stephanie Bennett; Louise Cardellina; T.C. Cherian, M.D.;
Rhoda Christopher; Una Fahy; Paula Fraser; Michael Harz; Sina Lee;
Thomas Lemens; Michael Lobel;
Barbara Miesch; Diane Neault; Sandra Rosado; Randy Shields; Gerald Paul Stone, Sc. Eng. D.;
Harold Wise, M.D.; and Sidney Zerinsky, M. Th., R.P.T., Ph.D.

Acknowledgments

Many thanks to the models who cooperated so patiently:
Cam Lorendo, Rochelle Sirota, John Burke, Madeleine Morel,
Paula Fraser, Lynette Mann, Jill Barber Petchesky, Rachel
Petchesky, Michael Macreading, Holly Wolf, Meg Wolf-Shapiro,
Jane Morgan, Jacqueline Carleton-Nathan, Steven Nathan,
Jennifer Paradine Carleton-Nathan, Suzie Brooks, Sabrina Brooks,
Dan Woldin, Louise Cardellina, Sharon Freedman and Noodge,
Wendy Spital, Tina Dudek, Antigone and Scott.

Thanks to the following people for their contributions:
Lanny Aldrich, Richard Schatzberg, Roger Mignon, Kathryn Greene, Amit Shah,
Maureen Charnis, Ed Caraeff, Nicholas Shrady, Antonio De Melo, Jerry Marshall
Virginia Rubel, Richard Amdur, Julianne Dobkin, Jo Irwin, Janice Johansen, Carolyn Barax

Special thanks to my editors:
To Jeannie Sakol for her brilliant insights, contributions and encouragement;
to Peter Skutches for his dedication in the early stages of the manuscript;
and to Melissa Smith, Paula Fraser, Sharon Freedman and Rhoda Christopher for their work.

I wish to express my great appreciation to T.C. Cherian, M.D.;
George Poll, D.C.; Alexander Teacher Jane Dorlester, C.S.W.,
Rhoda Christopher and Marjorie Conn, M.Th. & Ed.D., for helping to keep
my body and mind in good health throughout all the trials and
tribulations of writing and assembling this book.

Many thanks to those who were patient enough to
sacrifice many a massage in order for me to
complete this book.

Thanks to Michael Harz for his support and encouragement, and
for providing me with a place in the sun to do the writing.

Extra special thanks to Una Fahy for her creative photography and design,
and to Susan Margolis for her beautiful and precise illustrations.

An extra special thanks to Morey Antebi for helping me
in more ways than I can list.

Finally, I wish to express my gratitude to Harold Wise, M.D.;
Sidney S. Zerinsky, M.Th., R.P.T. & Ph.D. and Mary Marks, D.C.,
for reading and commenting upon my manuscript.

Table of Contents

Introduction

Massage is probably the oldest healing art in the world, having been rediscovered many times over the centuries. Today massage is regarded as a potent method of treating modern day stress, tension, emotional trauma and illness, replacing them with energy and vibrant health.

The Magic of Massage is a book whose time has come. Many books have been written about massage. Until now, none has sufficiently introduced and integrated the various systems so that the reader may learn to give and receive a nurturing, therapeutic and relaxing massage.

Ouida West's book takes the reader down the path to deeper awareness through the sense of touch, movement and energy.

Sidney S. Zerinsky, M.Th., R.P.T., Ph.D.
Clinical Director/Director of Faculty of the Swedish Institute Inc., School of Massage Therapy and Allied Health Sciences

Preface

I am pleased to be writing this preface to the second edition of *The Magic of Massage*. I sincerely hope that the techniques offered in this book will help to improve the quality of your health and your life in general. I also hope that the other sections will be helpful to you, especially the section in Chapter VI on Foods for Optimum Health.

Since the 1983 publication of this book my philosophy on massage has evolved but not changed significantly, while my philosophy on diet and life-styles has changed dramatically. I feel almost embarrassed each time I share my enlightenment because, in so doing, I am openly admitting that for almost thirty-eight years, without actually knowing it, I lived in a state of unawareness. I had always considered myself to be kind, responsive to any human being in need, respectful of animals and nature, conscious of not littering, against violence and war and supportive of equal rights for all human beings.

I remember, as a youngster, I would befriend and defend students who suffered the effects of crippling diseases, emotional disturbances or brain damage. If a child was harassed because she/he was "ugly" or fat, I would always encourage people to look into their hearts rather than at their faces or bodies. Likewise, I'd befriend and defend foreigners, blacks, Jews, French Canadians—any person who was considered too different to "fit in." I had always picked up, and found homes for, stray cats and dogs; I had also often paid veterinarians to treat injured birds or squirrels and, when they were healed, returned them to their natural habitat. I thought I was "doing my bit."

On April 20, 1985, my birthday, I was rudely awakened. I decided to reject the typical self-centered birthday activities and focus, instead, on a worthwhile cause outside myself. I considered attending a human rights or ecological rally, but by chance a poster led me to an animal rights rally. I imagined it would be interesting and informative, that I would probably join one of the organizations to show my support. I had absolutely no notion of the personal transformation I would undergo that day. What a shock! The animal rights rally forced me to realize that somehow I had successfully blocked from my consciousness all of the information on the suffering of animals: in factory farming, in laboratories, in hunting and fishing, in circuses, zoos and rodeos, and in the cosmetic industry. How could I have been so unaware? I suddenly realized I hadn't done nearly as much as I am capable of to help my animal friends. I was devastated; in quasi-ignorance I had betrayed them. I had not allowed myself to grasp the large-scale suffering and abuse of animals, undoubtedly because it was too painful to confront. I'm sure, too, that I was overwhelmed by a feeling of my own helplessness in improving their lot. I was sick from my guilt and their misery. I couldn't sleep or eat. I lost weight. I could hardly get to work . . . although once I was actually involved in giving a massage, I experienced some relief, probably because I felt I was in some way helping someone. For three months I was haunted by the cries of these abused animals, by their eyes filled with terror and confusion. I thought I would go mad; my feeling of helplessness was driving me to despair. And when I thought I could take no more, I became aware of other cries and other terrified, confused eyes—cries and eyes from all parts of the world; fellow humans suffering in pain, in hunger, in fear. I had also blocked human suffering from my conscious mind, because this, too, was too painful and confusing to confront. I was certain I would suffer a breakdown, that this added awareness was more than I could bear. Instead, though, it made me stronger. I realized that human beings were very often cruel not only to helpless animals but also to helpless children, women, and men. I also realized that only through total compassion, and dedication to a reverence for life, can humans become the highly evolved beings we must become in order to end these and all injustices.

At this moment I knew I would dedicate my life to ending human and animal suffering. Simultaneously, I also *fully realized* how close we have come to destroying the planet's ecology. I, like most people, had always been subliminally aware of these injustices, but I'd not brought them to a level of conscious awareness, no doubt because they were too depressing to confront. They are depressing, but they must be confronted. When I happened to overhear one woman say to another, "I decided to watch a documentary on ecological destruction last night, but it was so depressing that I turned the channel almost immediately," I realized I could no longer change my channel to avoid recognition of injustices—I heard and saw everything. I now know these harsh realities have made me stronger, in my commitment to the welfare of other human beings, to the rights of animals, to the rejuvenation of our planet's ecology. I am now driven, and gladly so, by this commitment. Although I still hear the cries and see the frightened, confused eyes, and am still aware of the planet's precarious ecological balance, these realities now act as a catalyst pushing me onward into action rather than reducing me to despair.

I began my personal overhaul by totally eliminating my use and consumption of all animal products. Then I started sending money and volunteering time to major organizations dedicated to fighting these injustices. I began to attend protests. I became a foster parent to two needy children. I modified my life-style, and continue to do so, to make it more basic and less extravagant. As a constant reminder of world hunger, one day a week and three weeks at the change of each season, I eat nothing but plain brown rice (or other whole grains) accompanied by one green and one yellow or orange vegetable at each meal, with no seasonings or oils. All these changes have certainly turned me around a few times, as well as upside down and inside out. The most surprising thing is that it hasn't been too difficult. I had always found change slow and painful, but it's not so slow or difficult when you know how important it is. To determine if an activity, action or thought moves me closer toward accomplishing my life's work, I need only imagine any or all of these injustices. Immediately and instinctively I know whether to stop or continue.

I am encouraging you to read what I have written here and in the section on Foods for Optimum Health with an open mind. What you think,

believe and *do* or don't do, does make a difference. I had always believed that there was nothing I could do to change these injustices except on a personal, one-to-one basis, but it's simply not true. Let me give you a perfect example. If women had not started fighting for women's rights in the nineteenth century by risking their security and even their lives, women today would still be living in miserable circumstances. We now have rights (although there are battles yet to be fought); we can live our lives more fully, thanks to those brave women and to all the women who persisted after them. Women have encountered great resistance from society in general in their quest for equality, and it was not only the uneducated who were unwilling to grant women equal rights. A highly respected Cambridge philosopher, Thomas Taylor, in a satirical publication refuting Mary Wollstonecraft's *A Vindication of the Rights of Women* proposed that if we were to give equal rights to women, then we would also have to give equal rights to animals! Philosophies can be made to change. You can and do make a difference, but you must realize that you may not witness the pinnacle of the change in your lifetime. That is not important; what is important is knowing that you dedicated your life to changing unjust situations. By adopting a vegetarian diet (or as close to vegetarian as possible) and philosophy you can contribute as an individual, on a minute-by-minute, day-by-day basis to the attainment of a peaceful cohabitation on earth. This diet and philosophy are also the only ways you can truly achieve the optimum health you seek.

Let these thoughts be a springboard for you into unexplored waters. Jump into the cold, refreshing waters of change. It's time to float downstream with life instead of swimming against the current. Be brave; change can be easy, and it is necessary, especially now. Our planet, human beings and other creature cohabitants cannot take much more abuse. The time has come for many, many more awakenings like mine. I sincerely hope you are next.

CHAPTER I

What Is Massage?

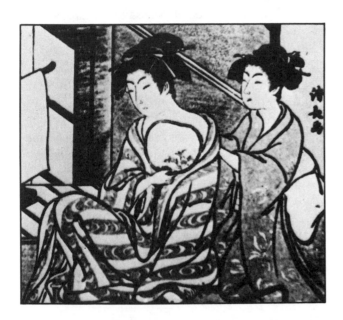 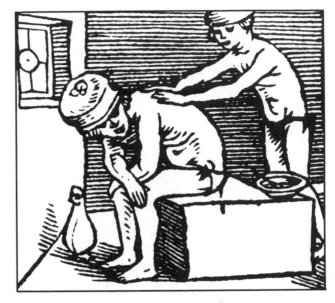

1) A BRIEF HISTORY OF EASTERN & WESTERN MASSAGE

The history of massage can be traced as far back as three thousand years before the birth of Christ. We can only speculate that humans prior to recorded history had an equally strong instinct to stroke or touch the body when it ailed, in order to console the afflicted, or speed up recovery. Even wild animals lick their wounds in an attempt to cleanse them and help them to heal. The following paragraphs briefly discuss all the major civilizations, beginning with the Chinese, that recognized and utilized the therapeutic benefits of massage.

The Chinese synthesized massage and gymnastics. Recorded history shows that the Orientals were using this form of massage at least three thousand years before the birth of Christ. A medical treatise known as the "Nei Ching," which is accredited to the Yellow Emperor Huang-Ti, contains the earliest Chinese references to massage. The Indian books of the Ayur Veda, written about 1800 B.C., refer to massage as rubbing and shampooing, which they recommend as a means of helping the body to heal itself. The medical litera-

ture of Egyptian, Persian and Japanese physicians makes many references to the benefits and usefulness of massage when attempting to cure or control numerous specific illnesses.

The Romans and Greeks, too, firmly believed in the benefits of massage. Homer, Herodotus, Hippocrates, Socrates and Plato, all among the greatest men of their times, all praised massage. Homer describes in *The Odyssey* the restorative powers for exhausted war heroes of rubdowns with oil. Herodotus states that massage can cure disease and preserve health, while Hippocrates, one of his pupils, believed that all physicians should be trained in massage. The writings of Plato and Socrates refer often to the use and excellent results of massage. Julius Caesar was pinched, i.e. massaged, everyday, because he suffered from neuralgia, and the famed Roman naturalist, Pliny, who was plagued by recurring asthma attacks, regularly received massage to help relieve these bouts. The Bible, too, contains innumerable references to the laying-on-of-hands as a method of healing the sick.

Massage continued to grow in popularity until the Middle Ages, at which time it lost its foothold in the medical profession because of a general atmosphere of contempt for the body and the physical world. Christianity placed an importance on the spiritual self that tended to exclude such earthly matters as the joy of physical well-being. All the sciences suffered great setbacks during this period of European history. Fortunately, the Renaissance brought back a renewed interest in the body and physical health. Much of the knowledge learned from the Eastern civilizations, as well as from the Greeks and Romans, was revived, and once again massage began to grow in popularity and develop as a science.

As the medical profession regained prestige, so too, did massage rise to new heights; for many prominent physicians incorporated massage into their approach towards curing the body and mind. Pare (1517-1590 A.D.) and Mercurialis (1530-1606 A.D.) were but two of the great physicians who integrated massage extensively into their medical practices. Ambroise Pare's methods proved to be so successful that he became the physician to four of France's kings. Mercurialis, a widely acclaimed Italian doctor, wrote a well-received treatise on massage and gymnastics that won him great fame and a rank among Italy's most prestigious physicians. The attending physician to Mary Queen of Scots led her to health in 1566 with his use of massage. Her condition was considered very grave and recovery was expected to be quite lengthy, but the doctor hastened her improvement through the application of massage techniques.

Massage took another great leap forward with the work of Per Henrik Ling. Ling, a native of Sweden, traveled to China and brought back some remarkably effective techniques of massage which he then assembled into a system known as "The Swedish Movement Treatment" or "The Ling System." There were many other physicians prior to and after Ling who contributed to the wealth of information now available on massage. Although they are too many to mention here in this brief history of massage, the bibliography lists numerous reference books which provide some

background in the history of massage. *Massage, Manipulation and Traction* by Sidney Licht, M.D., published by Robert E. Krieger Publishing Company, is one of the more detailed sources.

Currently, Swedish Massage and Japanese Shiatsu are the most popular methods of treating the body in Europe and on the North American continent. Shiatsu has recently been gaining a following of significance among practitioners and lay people. Even the medical profession is now beginning to take note of this intricate system of meridians and pressure points. There are many systems, some of which arose independently, currently in use in Europe and in North America, but the majority of them are off-shoots of either Swedish or Shiatsu. Some of the more popular independent and spin-off systems include: Rolfing, Soma Massage, Chiropractic, Touch For Health, Reflexology, Acupressure, Alexander Technique, Feldenkrais Method, Polarity and Barefoot Shiatsu.

2) THE MAGIC OF MASSAGE IS A GIFT

Massage seems magical because of the lack of scientific data explaining the body's complex systems, especially the meridian system. The magic lies, too, in the doer's ability to channel those mysterious life forces, that, when allowed to flow through us, make whatever we do more powerful and indeed quite magical. The Japanese speak of the hara as the place within the body where the essential energy of that body resides. It is in your hara, one-and-a-half inches below the navel, that you can find the magical strength to do what you are usually unable to accomplish. Don't be disturbed by the word *hara,* and don't worry if your knowledge of eastern philosophy is not comprehensive. Translated into lay terms, let your instincts be your guide. When you function on a purely instinctual basis, you are automatically in touch with those magical forces that allow you to sense things which normally escape your awareness. Instinct will usually, if heeded, guide you through many situations easily, gracefully and harmlessly. Apply the magic of those instincts to massage, and you will be able to sense where to touch, how to touch, and for how long in order to make your receivers feel better and even heal themselves.

The ability to give a magical massage without training or experience is a gift. Some people seem to be born with it. Most people, however, must learn how to give a magical massage. It may be learned more easily when one is desirous of mastering the art, and wishes to help someone feel better. Put your ego aside and listen to what the receiver's body is telling you. Let your instincts guide your hands as you fill your being with love and allow your compassion to flow from you to the receiver. If you are a clumsy person, do not despair. Massage from your hara, your center, and you too will be able to give a magical massage.

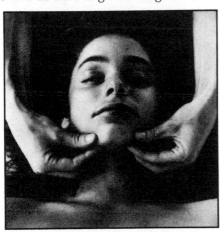

Massage is also a gift because you are giving your time to someone. You could just as easily choose to pursue a favorite pastime like playing tennis or watching television. Instead, you have chosen to spend a certain amount of your time giving of yourself to someone special or someone in need.

Massage is a gift in another way too. You, as the doer, are offering your receiver the gift of both physical and psychological health. It is a known fact that massage improves circulation of the blood and lymph, and that most conditions will improve if the circulation of these two vital fluids is encouraged. Therefore, while you are massaging your partner or friend, be fully aware of the benefits you are providing as you work.

Most of us do not get touched enough. Even though you may have an active sexual life, that does not mean you are receiving enough non-sexual touch. Experiencing massage by loving hands can help adults and children fulfill their needs for touch. Exchanging complete massages once a week or giving a quickie massage when it is needed helps to keep you feeling healthy and happy, as well as in touch with yourself and other human beings.

Finally, the ability to receive a massage is a gift, and many of us simply don't know how to accept a gift. It is often easier to give than to receive. The ability to let go and allow the doer to penetrate into your essential being to make you feel better must sometimes be learned. Not only is it the responsibility of the doer to make the massage successful, but also you, as the receiver, must help to make it work by allowing the doer to give.

The magic of massage is a gift in every sense of the word. If you are not one of the more fortunate people born with this gift, extend yourself and learn its magic so that massage can become an integral part of your life.

3) THE PSYCHOLOGY OF MASSAGE

Your state of mind when giving a massage is of utmost importance. Unless your feelings, awareness and motivation are unusually pure in nature, you will transmit your tensions to the receiver. If your tension levels are extremely high, chances are that your receiver will find the massage insensitive, indifferent or perhaps hostile. All life is composed of atoms. Atoms vibrate. The excitability of atoms is a known scientific fact, so watch your vibrations. If they are too rapid because of emotional upsets, either calm yourself or schedule the massage for another day.

If you are sick or feel like you might possibly be coming down with a cold or flu, do not give a massage. One obvious reason is that you may infect the receiver. Apart from that you must also realize that your energy level will be depleted. Not only will you run the risk of making yourself sicker, but also you will probably not be able to give a satisfying massage.

The most important rule to remember when giving a massage is to let your instincts be your guide. If you suddenly feel that you should touch a particular part of the body in a particular way, don't hesitate. Make a smooth transition from the technique you are presently implementing to that part of the receiver's body which is calling you, and employ the stroke or apply the pressure that is required to satisfy your instincts. Do not allow your ego to interfere while giving a massage because it will result in a less sensitive approach. Focus your mind on the receiver's tensions and fears, and watch them dissolve. Focus, coupled with your instincts, will enable you to feel the tension and fear hidden deep within the joints, muscles, organs and bones of the receiver. Imagine that you are a detective. Locate the assailant hiding in a joint, muscle, organ or bone, and dispose of the culprit.

It is not always easy to rid the body of its stored tension and/or fear. Once you locate a villain, try to coax it out by using the appropriate stroke or application of pressure. If you do not succeed after a reasonable amount of time, abandon your efforts for a while. Return to the area later, several times in one massage if necessary.

Humans tend to guard their tensions and fears as if they were precious jewels. Do not be overly aggressive when trying to dissipate them. Unwanted as these aspects of their psyche may be, most people are nevertheless reluctant to abandon any part of themselves. Allow love and compassion to come through your touch to show the receiver how much better the body will feel.

Many people attempt to bury tensions and fears within their bodies with the hope that the fears will remain a secret from themselves and the world. Though tensions may stay hidden for a while, they will eventually return in the form of bodily aches and pains. By this time the sufferer has no idea what the real problem is. A clever doer or massage therapist can communicate with these tensions and by compassionate manipulation can dissolve them. The doer may find it necessary to address the affected areas many times

before the tensions disappear. One aid in this process is praise. As you massage an affected area, utter words that will encourage the receiver to let go and to feel good. If you sense the slightest release, offer a compliment like, ''That was good! Now let's try for a little more.'' If the receiver releases all or a great deal of the tension and fear, exclaim, ''Oh that was beautiful! You really let that go!'' We all like to hear we're beautiful.

Many people have little idea where or to what degree they are holding their tension. Often they may believe they are relaxed, but you are confronted with rigid limbs. Don't criticize or try to force the receiver to admit to a tension the receiver may not be ready to accept. It's best to say, ''Oh, I think I've found some tension here. Let's see if we can work together to let it go.'' Often the person will relax further if you are encouraging, because the receiver will no longer feel threatened or alone in the struggle. When the receiver does release, don't forget the compliment.

The use of imagery is helpful in encouraging some people to release stored tensions and fears. Perhaps the image of a rag doll to suggest that they relax their limbs, or ask them to think about something that makes them feel happy and peaceful, like a ship at sea. You can even be sneaky, if you know the receiver well enough. Casually mention something you know makes the receiver feel good to drive away whatever worries that may presently preoccupy the receiver's mind.

Most people hide their misery in the same spots, most commonly in the neck, shoulders or lower back. Repeated recognition of these storage areas will help to discourage further build-ups and will thereby encourage a less tense and freer body and mind. One last caution to the doer, do not allow the negativism that is leaving the receiver's body to fill yours. As the tension is released, neutralize it and send it away from your finger tips into the atmosphere. Better yet, try to dissipate it outward even before it reaches your fingers. One method of neutralizing negative energy as it leaves the receiver's body is to visualize its transformation into something positive like a bouquet of wild flowers or a ray of sunlight or a fish swimming happily away.

CHAPTER II

Why Massage?

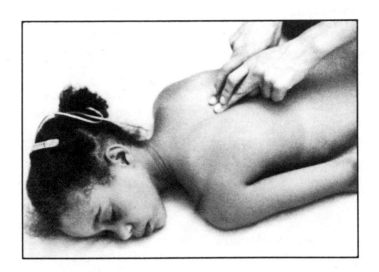

1) GENERAL REASONS TO MASSAGE

To massage or touch with the intention of relieving pain is an instinct basic to human nature. Since primitive times humans have touched and massaged themselves or others as the need has arisen. There are many instances, however, when it is more effective to touch a part of the body distant from the location of the pain. Our knowledge of distant-point therapy has been learned mostly through trial and error. Someone with a toothache, perhaps, accidentally hit the inner upper edge of the humerus bone on the same side as the aching tooth, and voila! The toothache disappeared. Likewise, someone with a headache may have received a blow to the outside of the thigh, midway between the hip and the knee, and the headache vanished. Discoveries like these were probably passed on by word of mouth from generation to generation. Eventually, though, they were recorded, and complex systems establishing the relationships between seemingly unrelated areas of the body evolved. The Chinese Acupuncture Meridian System and related disciplines which utilize distant-point therapy are discussed in Chapter III, Section 5 of this book.

When many Westerners think of massage, they think of health clubs or spas and a vigorous process of kneading, rubbing, pressing and slapping. Massage, however, can also be quiet, slow, penetrating and gentle. I define massage as any touch that is capable of evoking a change in the body. Even the lightest touch, when properly executed, may effectively stimulate circulation or alter the flow of energy within the body. Gentleness, as well as firm, penetrating pressure and a subtle, feathering motion, must also be considered valid massage techniques, for these methods have proven useful in relieving specific types of tension or pain. Massage, then, as the term is used in this book, refers to any type of touch.

Occasional massage treatments have been known to effect dramatic changes in both body and mind. However, to relieve or cure most physical and emotional problems, regular massage sessions are generally necessary. Based on my definition of massage as touch, I would like now to describe what massage, on a regular basis, can accomplish for your body and mind.

- Deep relaxation is induced by massage

- The release of tension in regular massage sessions often enables the receiver to overcome long-standing emotional turmoil because renewed energy becomes available to aid in coping with them

- Greater achievements are possible with renewed energy and a cleared mind

- Self-esteem improves

- The body and mind can be stimulated without the negative side-effects of caffeine or drugs

- Mental and physical fatigue is relieved

- Chronic neck and shoulder tension can be released

- Muscles receive an increased blood supply of nutrients that help to improve their functioning

- Calf cramps and other muscle spasms can be eliminated

- Waste products that accumulate in muscles after vigorous exercise can be removed to prevent soreness and aching

- Muscle tone can be improved, and muscular atrophy, due to forced inactivity, can be reduced

- Massage is a form of passive exercise that can partially compensate for lack of exercise

- Chest pains related to tight pectoralis muscles can be eliminated and a tension-causing fear of heart attack alleviated

- Fat stored in your tissues may be reduced

- Massage dilates blood vessels to improve circulation

- Arthritis patients experience relief because improved circulation to the joints reduces inflammation and pain

- Directly massaging the hands helps to relieve and sometimes eliminates neuralgic, arthritic and rheumatic disorders

- Bursitis responds favorably to massage

- Sprains heal more readily

- Fractures, breaks and dislocations take less time to heal

- Adhesions can be prevented or broken down to effect greater mobility

- The function of every internal organ can be improved, directly or indirectly, by the application of the many different techniques

- Digestion, assimilation and elimination can be improved

- The detoxifying function of the kidneys is increased

- Massage heightens tissue metabolism

- The lymphatic system is flushed by mechanically eliminating toxins and waste

- Massage returns blood to the heart thereby assisting in cardiac functions

- Massage can benefit anemics by increasing the number of red blood cells

- Eyesight and hearing can be improved

- Nasal congestion and sinus conditions improve dramatically and often totally disappear

- Sore throats can be encouraged to heal more quickly. If a sore throat is treated within the first hour, it can often be averted

- All types of headaches (Gall Bladder, Liver, Stomach, Large Intestine, emotional and migraine) can be eliminated

- The balding process can be stopped, reduced or reversed through frequent massaging of the shoulders, neck and head, and by making contact with the neuro-vascular holding points

- Wrinkles can be lessened due to improved circulation

- Back pain can be relieved

- Body fluid in the legs and arms can be reduced to decrease swelling and provide relief to tired or aching limbs

- Tired, burning, stinging or aching feet can be rejuvenated

❧❧❧❧❧❧❧❧❧❧❧❧❧❧❧

Massage is essential to your total good health. Unfortunately, most people consider massage a luxury. I disagree entirely, for everyone, regardless of age, will benefit from regular massage sessions. Given the daily pressures of the modern age, massage is a necessity. If you cannot massage yourself or exchange massages with a partner or friend, I recommend massage on a regular basis with a trained practitioner. If money is a problem, consider bartering services for massage sessions. Perhaps you could teach, baby-sit, or do light housekeeping in return for professional treatment. If you really want a massage, you can find a way to get it.

In any case, a basic understanding of massage is advantageous, because you will be able to help others or yourself when you least expect it and when it's needed most. One day when I was eating lunch in a restaurant, I heard a muffled scream from the kitchen. I peeked into the kitchen to see what had happened, and discovered the chef had cut her index finger. It was bleeding profusely. She bandaged it and managed to stop most of the bleeding, but the finger was throbbing. She found it difficult to continue working, and no one was there to relieve her. I asked if she would like me to stop the pain. She asked if I had an aspirin. "No," I said, "but I do know an acupuncture pressure point that will relieve the pain." Although she looked skeptical, she was desperate. I pressed firmly into her cheekbone, alongside the flare of her nose, for 60 seconds. When I released my pressure, the pain had stopped. She was startled, and looked at me as if I were a magician. I explained that the meridian or energy pathway for the large intestine begins near the base of the index fingernail, travels up the arm and over the shoulder, then up the neck onto the face, where it terminates next to the ala of the nose.

(See Meridian Illustration #3 on page 39.) It is possible to relieve pain that occurs at one end of the meridian by applying pressure at the other end. I instructed her to press the same terminal point, should the pain recur. When I returned to the restaurant several weeks later, the chef told me that her finger had begun to hurt a few hours after I had held the pressure point. She had then held the point herself for about one minute, and the pain had never again returned. She also mentioned that the finger had healed more quickly than usual. Evidently she cut her finger often, so she had many instances for comparison.

Another incident that proved acupuncture pressure points a valuable first-aid treatment occurred when I was walking on a beach one summer day. I witnessed a young guy punch another in the nose and walk away. The victim was lying on the sand and looking rather stunned when I reached him. I asked if he would like me to stop the pain and reduce the swelling of his left eye. "Why not," he muttered. I took the toe next to the big one and squeezed it for several minutes. In a few seconds the pain in his eye had begun to subside. At the end of three minutes the swelling had begun to go down. I instructed the fellow to squeeze the toe frequently for the next few days in order to help his eye to heal. I also suggested that he get some ice at the beach snack bar and apply it immediately to the swelling. He was too stunned to ask why pressure to the toe had alleviated the pain in his eye. It had worked because the stomach meridian begins under the eyes, travels down the face, neck, trunk and legs, and terminates near the nail of the second toe. (See (Meridian Illustration #1 on page 38.) Again, the meridian principle applies. If injury to the body occurs at a point near the beginning or end of a meridian, it can be treated by applying pressure to the acupuncture pressure point farthest from it on that meridian. (See the Meridian Chart on pages 38 and 39 for further possibilities.)

Massage seems a lot like magic, because you see something happen, but you don't quite understand why. Don't worry about not understanding why. Scientists will, no doubt, eventually be able to explain why acupuncture, acupuncture holding/

pressure points and allied practices are so remarkably effective. Until then, use the techniques and reap the benefits. Not only can massage greatly improve your physical and emotional well-being, but it also may enable you to help yourself and others cope with everyday tensions, many ailments and the unexpected injury.

2) WHY MASSAGE FOR COUPLES?

Chapter IV, How To Give A Complete 60-Minute Body Massage, is geared to partners or friends who want to give each other a thorough massage once a week. Partners who exchange massage on a regular basis inevitably develop a deeper, more meaningful relationship. As trust, understanding and communication improve, your partner becomes your friend as well as your lover.

Too many relationships are based primarily on sex. There comes a time, usually after a year, when the sexual passion in most relationships becomes less intense, less frequent and sometimes less satisfying. At this point many relationships go into a decline. Both parties begin to feel that they are no longer as sexually attractive or attracted to each other as they were before. Insecurities and rejection set in, and partners soon discover they can no longer communicate on any level. Relationships that are failing can usually be revived through regular massage because massage helps partners to put their problems, their emotional needs, their sexual desires, themselves and each other into proper perspective.

Massage can improve and heighten the sexual experience. For those who feel they already have a good sex life, massaging for ten to twenty minutes before sexual activity can heighten an already satisfying experience. Massage enhances sex with sensuality. The ability to be sensual can be learned, or re-learned. By massaging the non-sexual parts of the body, partners can express the depth of their feelings in a purely sensual fashion. Oils may be used to further enhance the pleasurable physical sensations of mutual stroking, feathering and kneading. The neuro-vascular holding

points for the sexual organs can also be wonderfully stimulating. Massage techniques can make a sex life fuller and more rewarding by bringing partners closer together before actual sexual gestures are made. Original techniques can be created too. Indeed, they will often evolve naturally, evoking equally free and natural responses.

Massage helps to release tension, re-establish communication and effect a flow of uninhibited expression between partners in a relationship, even after long periods of withdrawal and strain. Any number of circumstances can strain a relationship, and a tension headache is one of the most common. It takes only a few minutes, however, to release the blockages causing the headache. There are points that, when held, release anxiety and thus make it easier for a partner to cope with an emotionally charged situation and physical or psychological trauma. Repeated use of these points will help the partner to overcome shock more quickly and with less pain than usual, and will reduce the amount of tension found in the relationship.

A quickie massage, exchanged after a long hard day in the office or home, enables partners to enjoy the evening together. It frees them from the tensions of working in an office or looking after a family that can often become overpowering. Too many couples spend nights quarreling or complaining about how exhausted they feel. After the fifteen to twenty-five minutes it takes to exchange a quickie massage, they would feel refreshed and could enjoy an evening at home, go out to dinner, see a movie or visit a friend.

Massage can also be extremely useful during times of illness. When disease strikes a member of a couple, the other is often plagued by feelings of helplessness. The thought that there is nothing you can do to improve your loved one's condition is apt to make you sick and your partner sicker. Most illnesses can be improved, controlled or cured through the use of the correct pressure points and other massage techniques. Furthermore, if you and your partner massage each other while you are both still healthy, you will avert many unnecessary illnesses. The inclusion of regular massage exchanges in your weekly agenda will reward you, not only with fewer aches and pains, but also with more energy and enthusiasm. The two of you together will enjoy a generally improved state of health in body and in mind.

In short, massage is one of the nicest ways of saying "I Love You." No words need be spoken, for the offer of a massage, when your partner is feeling low or exhausted, says it all. It is a special kind of gift, a unique expression of yourself, your compassion and your love.

3) WHY MASSAGE YOUR CHILD?

Massage strengthens and solidifies the parent-child bond. Parents should begin massaging their child while it is still in the womb. All too often

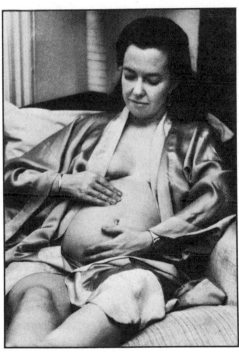

mothers have little physical contact with their child prior to delivery. Most mothers can locate the child's head at different times during the pregnancy and can determine whether the child is sleeping or awake, but too few of them spend enough time lightly touching and massaging the growing fetus through the abdominal wall. Massage helps the mother to understand and experience the child subliminally before it is born.

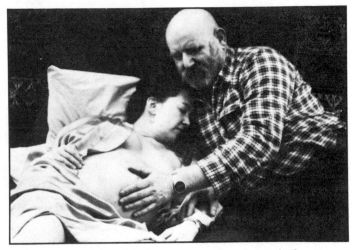

Fathers should also massage and touch the mother's abdominal area, although many only occasionally feel the baby while it is inside the womb. Frequent massage of the baby prior to birth helps the father to relate to the pregnancy experience and brings him closer to both the child and mother.

At the age of 5 or 6 a child usually begins to have the digital dexterity necessary to begin massaging their parents. Parents should encourage their child to do so. They should also be sure to respond with reassuring sighs and to offer the child compliments when a technique has been mastered. Too many children are brought up

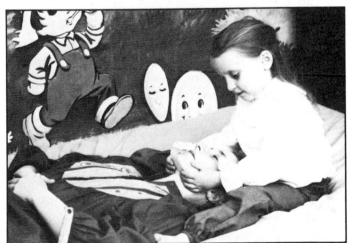

with little or no responsibility. As a result, they develop the attitude that whatever they need or desire will come to them with no effort on their part. Often they carry these unhealthy attitudes with them into adulthood. Massage is an excellent way to teach children that they can actively contribute to Mom and Dad's health and happiness.

19

Siblings, too, should be taught the techniques of massage. The more they exchange massages with each other, the better they will understand

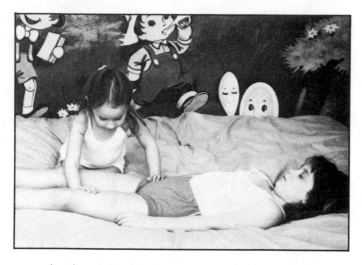

each other. Massage encourages sharing, which in turn promotes greater communication, builds trust and deepens the love between siblings, diminishing sibling rivalry.

Children, like adults, have physical and emotional complaints. When a child comes home after an upsetting day at school, what does a parent do instinctively to calm the child? Often a parent places the child's head in the hollow of the shoulder, then holds the back of the child's head or strokes the center of the child's back between the shoulder blades. The hollow of the adult's shoulder is touching the forehead frontal-eminence stress points of the child. The point on the back of the child's head corresponds to the adrenal glands, and contact there helps to relieve the tension produced by the upsetting events of the day. The neuro-lymphatic massage points for the emotional center of the brain are located in the center of the back. Intuitively the parent has touched all the correct points. The only problem is generally these points are not touched long enough or in a therapeutically effective way. Instead of giving a child an aspirin, parents should learn to stimulate the points that correspond to the child's complaints.

Minor illnesses respond quickly and easily to massage. With the knowledge gained from this book, a parent will be able to use massage and pressure points to bring about a speedy recovery in the child. Sore throats, colds, lung afflictions, earaches, toothaches, diarrhea and constipation are some of the common ailments that a parent can help a child overcome. Regular massage will also decrease a child's susceptibility to infections and improve the functioning of internal organs. It should also be remembered that children respond to massage much faster than most adults.

Equally important is the function of massage when a child is seriously ill and the parents, often totally frustrated, wish they could do something to help cure or improve the condition. This brings to mind the case of a newly married couple whose first baby was born with a hole in the heart. The doctors were uncertain as to whether the condition would improve. If it did, the doctors estimated it would take at least a year, and probably more. Frightened, helpless and miserable, the parents did not want simply to sit back and wait to see what would happen. Instead, they began using Touch for Health techniques to strengthen the baby's health. Within six months the hole had closed. The doctors were surprised, for they had never seen such a large hole close so quickly. The parents felt duly exultant, for they had helped to close the hole in their baby's heart. They had also turned agonizing months of helpless waiting into hopeful months of patient helping.

Massaging, holding or applying pressure to the points that correspond to a child's defective organ enables parents to feel helpful, and surely they are, for improved energy, blood and lymphatic circulation always helps an organ to function better and repair itself. It is understood, of course, that some illnesses are incurable; it is truly surprising to discover that most conditions can be improved through correct stimulation of the points associated with the organ involved.

Regular massage also helps a child to mature more readily and cope more effectively with social pressures and expectations. Children who grow up receiving massage tend not to experience major behavioral problems. And the severity of pre-existing behavioral problems for those children who did not receive massage throughout childhood may be lessened by beginning a regular massage program. Furthermore, massage can improve a child's perception of depth, thickness, texture and shape, in order to develop perceptive abilities at an age earlier than the childhood norm. Touch and massage can increase a child's I.Q., and what parent would not want a more intelligent daughter or son?

4) WHY SELF-MASSAGE?

Self-massage is infrequently utilized and greatly misunderstood. Most people have never heard of it, and those who have do not understand the extent of its benefits. Self-massage enhances an understanding of the body, and thus enables you to interpret your body signals with greater skill. The ability to translate your body signals into bodily needs can correct a disturbance long before it develops into a serious illness and can save you much pain and suffering.

Self-massage is a must for everyone. It is useful at any age, but self-help through massage is especially rewarding for older people who live alone. There will always be times when you need a massage and no one is available to administer it. Even if you live with someone, you will not always feel free to ask your partner for help. With the knowledge you obtain from this book, you can improve your physical health and psychological well-being.

Your health may benefit in many ways through self-massage. It can release blockages to improve the flow of your vital energies. It will develop your awareness of your skeletal and muscular systems enabling you to increase flexibility, and revitalize your constitution. The more you

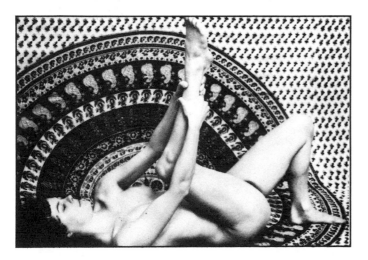

learn about your body through self-massage, the greater your ability will be to improve its condition, and keep illness and pain out of your life.

Utilization of the proper points at the correct times can improve organic functions. To improve digestion, for example, you should do the stomach, pancreas, liver, gall bladder and small intestine points before and after meals. If you have just indulged in a greasy meal, by massaging the liver and gall bladder points you can help your body cope with the excess intake of fat. Don't fool yourself, however; fatty and fried foods are harmful. Do not assume that by assisting your liver and gall bladder each time you eat a fatty meal, you can undo all harm. This advice is meant to help you through only an occasional cheat. Self-massage can also be utilized to help organs that are not operating efficiently, as in cases of diabetes, heart problems or a weak bladder. By stimulating the correct points several times daily, you can vastly improve the function of the affected organ.

Take time to help your body. There are many ways you can help your vital organs. Let's say you're painting your house and the paint fumes become rather overpowering. It would make good sense, and provide relief, if you massaged your lung lymphatic points. Your liver, too, could use some assistance in coping with the extra load of toxins. You could also massage general circulation points.

Help is only as far away as your own hands in the event of household accidents. Should you hit your thumb with a hammer, you would instinctively hold it, squeeze it or suck on it. Such measures would make your thumb feel a little better, but an understanding of meridians, or energy pathways, would enable you to handle the accident more effectively. You would know that the lung meridian ends in your thumb, and that by pressing and massaging the origin of this meridian, which is located in the chest near the shoulder, you could relieve the pain and help your thumb to heal faster.

Self-massage also helps to firm or build up the muscles of your body. You can tone or develop major muscles of your body by using the corresponding points for the muscles you wish to improve. By doing the points before and after you exercise, you can alert your body and brain to which muscles in particular you want to shape up.

If you often feel tired and lacking in energy, stimulation of your adrenal and brain points will provide a quick, safe pick-me-up. The energy boost you receive from massage, unlike caffeine and drugs, has no harmful side-effects. If, on the other hand, you are having trouble sleeping at night, sedation of your adrenal glands and holding your frontal eminence points will induce sleep in five minutes. Dangerous over-the-counter drugs are unnecessary.

Self-massage techniques will enable you to overcome tension instead of allowing it to overcome you. Traumatic events will no longer shatter you physically and emotionally. A telephone call bringing bad news, for instance, does not have to be debilitating. You probably have noticed many people place their hands on their foreheads in times of great stress. You have probably done it yourself. The neuro-vascular holding points that connect to the emotional center in the brain are located on the frontal eminence of the forehead. More by instinct than knowledge, you try to touch these correct holding points. With knowledge as well as instinct, however, you hold these points correctly and for the necessary length of time. The intensity of the traumatic experience would diminish, and you would become calmer, more rational and better able to cope. Some types of depression can also be controlled by utilizing the frontal eminence neuro-vascular holding points on a regular basis. Generally, self-massage can prevent accumulated daily psychological stresses from developing into a serious physical or emotional illness.

If you are extremely busy and don't have the time for self-massage, try incorporating some of the techniques into each day's shower or bath. By the end of one week you will have stimulated all your major organs. Your body will be grateful for the extra help. It has a big job coping with all the tension and toxins in the world today.

Many people tell me that self-massage is not as satisfying as being massaged by someone else,

and so why bother? Well, I can't deny it. Lying down for one hour and receiving a massage is far more pleasant than having to do it yourself. Nevertheless, some physical manipulation is preferable to none, as is feeling healthy and fit to being sickly and tired. No one knows your body as well as you. With some knowledge of massage and your instincts as your guide, you will know better than anyone else where and how you need to be touched. You will also know how much pressure to apply without causing pain. Much of the feeling of pain is really fear of pain. When you are in control of the pressure, you eliminate the fear and can therefore press harder than a massage therapist might. In some instances, increased pressure brings faster and greater relief. Remember, too, that once the mechanical process of learning the techniques is accomplished, you are free to focus on the sensations emanating from the point of contact and to increase the pleasures of self-massage.

Massaging yourself is a very positive statement. You love yourself. You think you deserve the time and attention, and you give it to yourself. While it seems natural and right to help others, caring for oneself seems somehow indulgent. We have been conditioned from childhood to believe that being good to ourselves is wrong. Loving ourselves is considered a worse offense. It's time to stop perpetuating this fallacy. If you can't be good to yourself, how can someone else be good to you! If you don't love yourself, who will love you? Finding and keeping love or friendship begins with you and your ability to love yourself, and then with your capacity to love someone else.

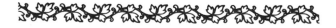

5) WHY MASSAGE YOUR PET?

Since the beginning of recorded history, humans have had pets. There is also anthropological evidence to suggest that pets were equally common in prehistoric communities. Why have humans always had pets? What are the reasons for creature companionship, when most people are looking avidly for human companions? Why are pets, especially dogs, called our best friends?

Pets are terrific companions. They are easy to please, basically self-sufficient, relatively uncomplicated, essentially happy by nature and almost always ready to communicate. Pets aren't critical or judgmental, and they don't care if you are famous or poor. Pets love you, regardless of how you feel or look. They listen to you when you ramble and reach out to you when you are feeling low. They are patient. If you come home late, a pet won't scold or cross-examine you. Instead, it will be loving and happy to see you. Pets only want to love and be loved. Although I am referring largely to cats and dogs, most pets possess these attributes.

Pets have also served humans in many ways. Eskimos could not survive without their sled dogs. Saint Bernards have saved many a life. Some dogs are protectors, while others act as eyes or ears for the unfortunately handicapped. Cats are useful as rat and mouse exterminators. The list of services rendered to humans by animals is endless, but animals generally serve humans because we train them to do so. They would undoubtedly prefer to be free. Massaging them is a wonderful way to show your appreciation for their lifetime commitment.

The most important aspect of the bond between humans and pets is the exchange of friendship and love. All humans need some form of physical contact in order to live a relatively happy, healthy life. Leading psychologists have recently stated that humans require at least twelve hugs a day for optimum health and happiness. Not all of us are fortunate enough to have a human companion to hug. Hugging a pet achieves similar results. If you hug or pet your animal friend twelve times a day, both of you will become healthier.

Regularly massaging your pet strengthens the bond of friendship and love that already exists between the two of you. The more energy and time you invest in strengthening this bond, the greater your returns. You will be rewarded with a more happy, playful, alert, intelligent, responsive, protective and loving pet. To elicit these results, an occasional pat on the head is not enough. Regular massage is required.

Pets pick up human tensions. If you are upset or angry, your pet will become very nervous or insecure. Your pet may feel itself the cause of your dissatisfactions. Whatever the pet may feel, it's important for you to realize that your best friend is going through your hard times with you. It is, therefore, only fair for you to massage your pet in order to help release the tension it has absorbed

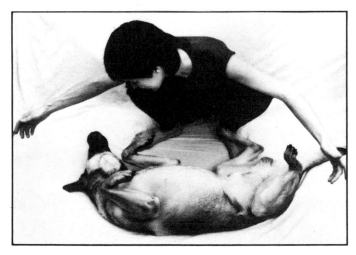

from you. Remember, your pet would probably feel happy or enthusiastic most of the time, if you felt that way too. Finally, it is also therapeutic for *you* to massage your pet. Recent studies indicate that people who have pets are less likely to have heart attacks.

If you have a pet that is frightened or aloof, massage can help restore its trust in you. You may not have caused your pet to be distrustful. Somewhere, someone, perhaps previous owners or thoughtless children, did the damage, but you can undo it. The more you massage and talk to your pet, the more friendly and trusting it will become.

One last important consideration is that massage is a form of passive exercise. If your pet cannot get outdoors to play and run, massage at least partially compensates for this lack. Older people should find this particularly helpful, as it is often difficult for them, because of physical handicaps, to assure their pets proper exercise. Massage will improve your pet's circulation, protect it against muscular atrophy, discourage premature illness and generally encourage a state of well-being.

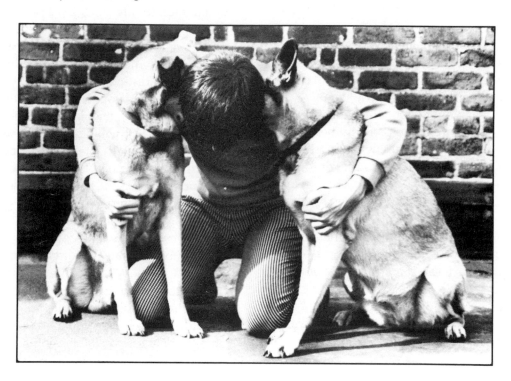

CHAPTER III

What You Need To Know For Best Results

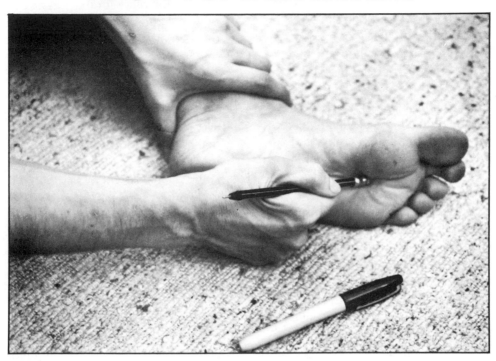

1) PREPARATIONS & ACCESSORIES

a) GENERAL PREPARATIONS & ACCESSORIES

Silence your telephone. If the telephone rings while you are receiving a massage, it will jangle your nervous system. It will wake you if you are sleeping and interrupt your flow of communication if you are not. Take your phone off the hook, or else turn down the ring and either cover the phone with a pillow or put it into a dresser drawer or closet. If you have an answering machine, switch it on and turn down all volume settings. If you have a jack, unplug it. Do as you please, but be sure to take care of this important matter. During massage, the telephone is an unwelcome intrusion.

Do not disturb. Place a "do not disturb" sign on your door to discourage unexpected visits from friends or neighbors. On it state the time you will be available, and if you have a doorman, tell him during which hours you will *not* be receiving. The time you set aside for massage is special. Do not allow interruptions.

Turn off glaring lights. Subtle lighting is a must. Bright lights strain the eyes and make it difficult to relax. When you become experienced at massage, try doing it in the dark. Without your eyesight your sense of touch becomes much more acute.

Control temperature. Air-conditioning is fine for the doer during the summer months. The receiver, however, will probably feel cold, as body temperature drops during a massage. A fan directed at the doer is ideal, for its breeze will only indirectly reach the receiver and will be deflected enough not to cause a chill. In the winter, when additional heat is required, do not use a space heater. Its intense heat can make the doer faint. Also, one part of the receiver's body is likely to be burning hot and the rest uncomfortably chilled.

An electric heater is dangerous because sheets, carpets and even flesh can easily be burned. Use an electric blanket whenever the receiver is likely to be cold. A receiver who feels chilled or cold will become tense and find the massage most unpleasant. Neither receiver nor doer benefits from a discomforting massage. If the doer exposes only the part of the body being massaged, the receiver will remain warm, relaxed and secure under the electric blanket.

Control drafts. A slight draft is harmless to the doer, but it can be quite chilling to the receiver. Drafts decrease the pleasure of the massage, diminish its benefits and can cause stiff or cramped muscles.

Incense creates a relaxing atmosphere . If you enjoy the fragrance of burning incense, use it. If, however, you start to sneeze, you may be allergic to it. Teary eyes and difficulty breathing are also allergic reactions. Incense is not essential, but the fragrance is conducive to relaxation and enjoyment.

Massage on a mat on the floor. A 1½-inch foam mat covered with a sheet is ideal, but if you do not want to invest in a mat, the blanket method is adequate. If one of your floors is padded and carpeted, all you need is two blankets. Fold each blanket into thirds. Stack one on top of the other. Spread a sheet over the blankets, and you've got it. Two blankets, stacked on a carpeted and padded floor, usually provide enough padding for the receiver's back and enough cushioning for the doer's knees. Remember, if the doer is not comfortable, that discomfort is transmitted to the receiver, and the pleasure and benefits are diminished for both. Do not give a massage on a mattress or futon. Instead of penetrating the receiver, most of the force of your pressure will be absorbed by the mattress. Furthermore, the receiver will become increasingly more conscious of the doer's every move, and the massage itself will become rocky and distracting. It is also quite easy for the doer to fall onto the receiver, as it is difficult to keep your balance on a mattress.

Prepare an extra blanket. If you do not own an electric blanket, keep a soft blanket handy in the event that the receiver gets cold. For some people a sheet is sufficient, but most require a blanket for

warmth part way through the massage. If the room can't be adequately heated, you may need two blankets for the receiver. Fold each blanket in four. Cover the receiver's torso with one blanket, and use the other for the legs and feet. Expose only that part of the body you are massaging in order to guarantee the receiver's comfort.

For the sake of clarity all photographs depict the receiver under ideal temperature conditions, thereby rendering a sheet or cover unnecessary.

Music soothes and relaxes. Music played softly in the background encourages relaxation. Loud music, however, distracts rather than soothes. Excellent selections of music, recorded for the express purpose of relaxing overly stimulated nervous systems, are available on tape. Some people find recordings of sea sounds particularly effective. Others prefer tapes of bird calls, which can lull the receiver's mind with the tranquil sounds of the country on a bright sunny day. I don't advise listening to music that is accompanied by lyrics, because lyrics tend to keep the mind focused rather than allowing it to free-associate. Select the music of your choice, and have the tapes or records ready to be played prior to beginning the massage. See page 188 for suggestions on the purchase of appropriate music.

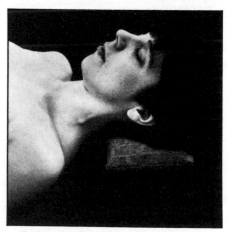

Raise the head with a pillow.

Raise the head with a pillow. Place a thin 1 to 2 inch pillow under the receiver's head. When the receiver is lying in the supine position, the head tilts back slightly and pinches the first few cervical vertebrae. Elevation of the head releases this pressure from the affected vertebrae. It thereby encourages the body to relax more readily and to be more receptive to the benefits of massage. If you don't have a thin pillow, use a towel folded several times. Prepare the pillow or towel prior to beginning the massage, and keep it within easy reach so that you can insert it without any distraction under the receiver's head.

Raise the receiver's legs while lying supine and prone. Place one folded bed pillow under each

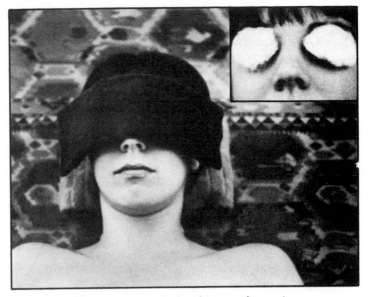

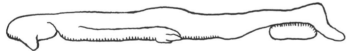

of the receiver's legs. Lying flat on the back puts a strain on the lower back. Since the receiver is supine during more than half the massage, low back strain or pain can easily result. People who suffer from back pain will almost always develop some discomfort during the massage if their legs are not raised. Even those who don't will find that their lower back begins to ache from lying supine too long. Raising the legs reduces the arch of the lower back and thus removes the strain on the muscles of the lower back. Use the same pillows

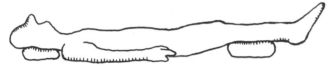

under the ankles while the receiver is lying prone. Not only will back tension be lessened, but also the feet will rest more comfortably on the mat.

Relieve eye-strain. Place cotton balls soaked in witch hazel, or in a cold solution of the herb eyebright, over the closed eyes. Drape a folded towel over the eyes and forehead. The folded towel serves both to cover the frontal eminence tension points and to keep the cotton balls in place. If you prefer to use eyebright, which can be purchased in most health food stores, prepare the solution by steeping one teaspoon of the herb in one cup of

boiling water, covered, for three to five mintues. Use only a fresh solution of eyebright. Refrigeration keeps a solution of eyebright fresh for two to three days. Chill the eyebright or witch hazel prior to application. Be sure to state that you are placing cold cotton balls over the eyes in order to prepare the receiver for the cold sensation.

Oil the back. You may use a small amount of oil on the back prior to beginning Back Technique #4, which is described in Chapter IV. It is not necessary, although some people feel a massage is incomplete unless they are oiled. In any case, use the oil sparingly. Work it well into the skin with upward or downward long, stroking motions. The back must not be oily or slippery when you begin Technique #4. Do not use oil on any other part of the body, as oiling interferes with pressure techniques. Massaging oil into the back does help to release some of the superficial tension stored in the muscles. This stroking motion, known as effleurage, also significantly improves venous and lymph circulation. The following oils are excellent: coconut, safflower, sesame, olive and almond, or any combination of these.

Remove jewelry. Jewelry can interfere with massaging techniques by scratching the receiver's skin. As this would be an unexpected, unpleasant and unwelcome experience for the receiver, play it safe by removing bracelets, watches and rings.

Short finger nails are important. Nails that extend beyond the tips of the fingers are too long for comfortable massage.

Clean hands are a must. As you will be touching the receiver's eyes and your fingers will be in the receiver's ears, clean hands are an absolute MUST. Many unpleasant conditions can be communicated via the hands. To avoid the possibility of any embarrassing situations, begin every massage with freshly washed hands and well-scrubbed nails. Clean hands also allow for greater sensitivity.

To be or not to be nude? If you are massaging your lover, it is sometimes very nice to be nude along with your partner. The reason is not at all sexual. Removing the clothing barrier allows both of you to relax more readily. Equally exposed and vulnerable, you can more easily share the intimacy of massage and achieve a feeling of oneness.

Wear loose clothing. Tight pants or shirts will make your experience as the doer most unpleasant. Avoid cutting off the circulation to any part of the body by wearing loose, comfortable clothing.

Don't forget the cold water wash. After completing a massage, it is an excellent idea to rub your hands together vigorously under *cold* water and allow the water to run from above your elbows down your forearm. Any negative energy that may have seeped from the receiver's body into your hands can be released in this manner. You will feel the difference, and you will also prevent unwanted energy from entering your body.

b) SPECIAL CONSIDERATIONS FOR MASSAGING CHILDREN

Draft & temperature control are especially important for young infants and children. If the possiblity exists for the child to experience a chill, massage the child in soft, loose, comfortable clothing.

Children new to massage are sometimes fidgety. Until the child adjusts to being handled in this manner, a teddy bear or soft cuddly friend will help. Initially, the child will fondle the toy, but will soon ignore it and enjoy the massage.

c) SPECIAL CONSIDERATIONS FOR SELF-MASSAGE

Tools can help. A ball point pen with an eraser or a thick marker pen with a rounded end can be useful when massaging the bottom of the foot. Unless your thumbs are exceptionally strong, they may tire or ache. These tools will enable you to apply firm pressure and experience maximum

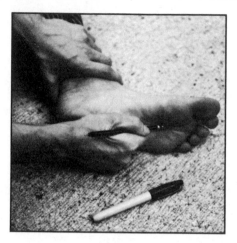

penetration with the least effort. Keep your tools clean. Your natural oils, as they accumulate on the tools, can make it dangerous, because your grip may slip while you are applying pressure. The result could be a painful experience. If you don't like the idea of using a foreign object, alternately use your thumbs and knuckles to apply pressure.

Loofa sponge. If you massage yourself in the tub or like to take a bath immediately after a massage, a loofa sponge rub is a great way both to end your massage and to improve circulation.

Pillows. Keep several pillows handy. You may need one or more of the pillows to help you assume a position comfortably.

d) SPECIAL CONSIDERATIONS FOR MASSAGING YOUR PET

When to begin massaging your pet? Do not attempt to massage your pet when it is spirited or excited. This is the time to play with your pet. When your pet is relaxed or sleeping is the best time to begin its massage. Be careful, however, for a sleeping animal can easily be startled by an unexpected touch. Speak gently to your pet just prior to touching it, so that the pet is aware of your approach.

Where to begin massaging your pet? Always begin by massaging the pet's favorite spots, which may be behind the ears, on the belly or under the chin. Once you have the pet under your loving control, you are free to begin implementing other techniques.

Introduce new techniques gently and slowly, so as not to alarm the pet and to enable it to adjust. Don't make sudden changes from one technique to the next. If you make the transition gradually, your pet will remain relaxed, receptive and quiet as you introduce each new procedure.

Keep your hands on your pet at all times. Some pets will suddenly jump up if you remove all contact. To avoid having to calm your pet several times throughout the massage, keep in touch.

Never force your pet into an unnatural position. Animals often feel trapped if they are forced into positions unnatural to them. Let your pet assume its own comfortable position and work from there. Some pets are more flexible than others. Stretches and rotations should be attempted only with loose, relaxed animals. Regular massage, however, will usually improve the flexibility of the most rigid limbs and will enable you gradually to introduce stretching and rotation.

e) SPECIAL CONSIDERATIONS FOR A QUICKIE MASSAGE

Spread a sheet on a carpeted and padded floor, turn down the telephone, dim the lights, and begin. Perhaps you have switched on some soothing music to help release tension, and the receiver may have undressed. Neither music nor nudity, however, is essential for a quickie massage. Time is. In Japan many people enjoy the refreshment of a Shiatsu massage during a lunch break, when time is obviously limited. A quickie massage can change the mind of any partner or friend who says, "I just can't go out tonight, I'm too tired." It will take you 15-25 minutes to convince your partner otherwise, for that is how quickly the Magic of Massage works.

2) PROPER FRAME OF MIND FACILITATES MOVEMENT OF BODY ENERGIES

Set all worries and thoughts aside. Remember that a worried or preoccupied mind cannot give the all that is necessary for a magical and therapeutically effective massage. The receiver will undoubtedly benefit to some degree from an absent-mindedly administered massage, but why settle for less? If you're going to give a massage, give it. Be there.

If you are one of those people who doesn't feel quite right unless your mind is active with worry or thought, try thinking about helping the receiver to relax and enjoy the massage. You can worry in double time, once the massage is over. Chances are greater, however, that after a few weeks of giving and receiving massage, you won't feel quite so compelled to worry. Massage on a regular basis does wonders for compulsive worriers, because the magic of massage calms not only the body but also the mind.

Keep your mind free and clear from mundane thoughts. While some people are given to excessive worry and gnawing anxiety, others are plagued by the trivial and mundane. Free your mind of lists and chores, of shopping or laundry that must be done, of floors that need washing, of lawns that should have been cut last week. Be there, with the receiver and the massage. An uncluttered mind effects a better massage.

Fill your mind and body with caring and compassion. At least fifty percent of the success of massage is determined by how much you, as the doer, want to help. Your only concern should be the well-being of the receiver. Your compassion will encourage the receiver to release tension and to enjoy a far more effective massage. What you give is reflected in what you receive. If your mind is focused exclusively on the receiver, you will drop your defenses and magically share in the benefits of the massage along with the receiver.

Breathing is important. When massaging yourself or someone else, allow yourself at least one minute before beginning the massage to regulate your breathing. Slower and slightly deeper than normal breaths will put you in touch with the "now" of the experience and will enable you to give a more effective massage. Do not inhale or exhale so deeply that breathing becomes an effort. Deep, but relaxed breathing is the secret. Don't force huge quantities of air into or out of your lungs. Simply inhale completely, then exhale completely. Little by little you will begin to relax. The depth of your inhalations and exhalations will automatically increase, because your diaphragm will have become more and more relaxed. Focus on your breathing. Focused breathing quiets the body and mind at the same time that it increases awareness of physical sensations. Deep breathing also oxygenates the blood. A body that is deprived of its fair share of oxygen experiences fatigue more rapidly than one accustomed to the rewards of deep breathing. Unfortunately, most of us are shallow breathers, as foul-smelling air, coupled with tension, discourages full breathing. Over a period of years, however, shallow breathing only intensifies that tension and increases the chances of illness. So, remain subliminally focused on your breathing pattern. Keep it slow and a little deeper than usual.

Keep your body relaxed. If your body is not relaxed while you massage, you will become tired and tense. You won't enjoy the experience, nor will the receiver. Consequently, both of you may shy away from the routine of massage. Hang loose! Giving a massage should be a pleasant experience. Allow your head to float freely on your neck, and keep your shoulders relaxed, not tense and raised up to your ears. Keep your back as straight as possible and free from abnormal con-

cave or convex curves. Make frequent mental checks to maintain your relaxed posture.

Know what you are massaging. Do not think of massage as an application of pressure only to the skin. You want to reach the core of the receiver. Think penetration—penetration to the bones' very marrow, to the vital centers of the organs and to the core of the nervous system. Be aware that to penetrate does not mean to cause pain. Focus your attention on the point of contact. What does it feel like? Is the point soft, hard, hot, cold, raised, hollow, active or dead? Do you feel energy radiating from the pressure point? Allow your instincts to dictate how much pressure to apply.

What is the receiver's frame of mind? The receiver should also focus attention on the pressure applied to each point. Focusing on the contact points helps to keep the receiver's mind free of extraneous worries and thoughts. This kind of concentration will often induce the receiver to fall asleep very soon after the beginning of the massage. The receiver must be submissive, must allow the doer to penetrate to the very core of her/his being. Above all, the receiver must be willing to receive the magic of massage.

Focus your attention. If the pressure point or massage technique corresponds to a particular organ, focus your attention on that organ. Try to imagine the organ's location in the body, and try to visualize its shape and size. With a little practice, thorough concentration and a lot of desire, both the receiver and the doer will be able to feel the energy moving into and through the organ being dealt with. Furthermore, the energy, blood and nutrients will reach their destination with greater ease when you focus your attention.

Execute Penetration with slow, sure strokes. Once you have made contact with a pressure point, penetration must be slow and easy. Never poke or dig unexpectedly into the receiver. When applying pressure, begin very gently and gradually increase your pressure to approximately half the receiver's capacity. When you are certain the receiver is comfortable, slowly proceed to apply the remainder of the pressure. Massage and pressure techniques must be executed with patience and without haste. Fast or energetic movements will jar the receiver out of the placid state you have worked so hard to achieve. Remember, your aim is to relax and soothe. As your confidence, or lack of it, will be picked up intuitively by the receiver, work slowly, easily and surely.

Establish a regular rhythm. A predictable rhythm calms the mind and relaxes the body. The application of pressure or massage in a hypnotically repetitive rhythm disposes the mind to ignore all but what is being done to the body. Keep your rhythms slow, as fast rhythms fail to relax effectively. A slow, predictable rhythm will also facilitate the movement of body energies.

Close your eyes. By closing your eyes, you eliminate your sense of sight and heighten your sense of touch. The more intense your touch, the more compassionate and magical will be your massage. Until recently, all practitioners of massage in Japan were blind. Not only did this marvelous custom create work and a meaningful existence for blind individuals, but also the receivers experienced an extraordinarily sensitive and compassionate massage.

Music calms the mind. If it is difficult for you to achieve the proper frame of mind for massage, music can be a useful tool to calm and soothe the mind. Choose music that both you and the receiver enjoy, though classical, jazz or cosmic sounds are most conducive to massage. Tapes are better than records. Tapes can easily be reversed with one hand, while the other remains in constant contact with the receiver. Keep the tape recorder close at hand, so that you don't have to break this contact. If possible, record some of your favorite music on a 45-minute tape. Tapes offering forty-five mintues of cosmic sounds are available especially for massage. Music without lyrics is preferable, and keep the volume low. Music should enhance and complement the massage, not dominate it.

Chanting clears your mind and relaxes your body. If you don't have tapes or records suitable for massage, chanting can effectively clear your mind and relax your body. If you don't know how to chant, hum random notes. Do not feel inhibited. Let your instincts dictate whether you should hum a low or high note. Begin humming the note

immediately after you have inhaled deeply, and continue it as long as you can exhale comfortably. The sound and vibration of the hum should come from the abdomen or lower chest, not from the throat, mouth or nose. If the sounds and vibrations emanate from these upper regions of your body, you are tense and need to make a conscious effort to relax and lower the hum to the abdominal area. Don't hum a familiar tune, as it will bring intrusive associations to mind. The notes you hum should be random and inspirational. Let them reflect your feelings and needs. Vary the pitch and duration of each sound. Chanting can create a strong feeling of oneness between you and the receiver that will encourage the release of energy and increase the benefits of massage.

Prepare for unexpected disturbances.
If you have attended to all the preparations and accessories listed in this section of the book, you will begin the massage calm, relaxed and confident. Sensing your readiness, the receiver will more easily submit to your touch and the magic of massage.

Proper frame of mind for self-massage. In self-massage you are both the doer and the receiver. As the doer, you must learn to function without much thought or effort. Several practice massages should enable you to master the techniques sufficiently, and the actual doing of the massage will cease to command your attention. As the receiver, you are primarily the experiencer. Focus your attention more on the physical sensations of your self-massage than on its technical execution. The more conscious you are of sensual responses, the greater will be your pleasure and the more fully realized your benefits. Practice makes perfect. Self-massage can be almost as rewarding and fulfilling as being massaged by someone else, if you maintain the proper frame of mind and allow the magic of massage to flow through your hands.

Learn to develop X-ray vision. Study the anatomical diagrams. (Terminology is irrelevant.)Then close your eyes and try to visualize them in detail. Practice this frequently, five minutes at a time. Soon you will be able to see into the body you are massaging. (If possible, study a skeleton to improve the three dimensionality of your vision.)

3) HOW TO GIVE A MASSAGE WITHOUT FEELING FATIGUED

It's easy to give a massage without feeling fatigued by the process. You simply have to know the tricks of the trade. These tricks or rules can be applied to all massage, be it massage for children, the family pet, someone else or yourself. It will require some discipline, at first, to learn the tricks, but if you practice them assiduously and keep regular check on yourself, you will soon be subconsciously assuming the correct posture, positioning and angle of penetration. Without effort you will be allowing the magic of massage to flow without interruption.

Assume the correct posture for the technique you are using. Be sure to study the photographs and text accompanying each technique. Try to assume exactly the posture shown in the photographs or described in the text. These postures are time-tested and offer maximum comfort for most people. If for some reason you are unable to assume the recommended posture, work out one that is comfortable and practical for you. Keep in mind, however, that you must not be hunched while you work. Try also to position yourself so that you are perpendicular to the surface to which you are applying pressure.

Comfort is of utmost importance. If at any time your position ceases to be comfortable, you must alter your posture. Otherwise, your discomfort will be transmitted to the receiver, and the massage will be a less pleasurable experience for both of you. The trick is to change positions without disturbing the receiver. NEVER move suddenly or jump up quickly. And do not take your hands off the receiver's body while trying to assume a different, more comfortable position. Abrupt and disruptive movements break down the bond between the doer and receiver, and five or six such disturbances could defeat the purpose of the massage. Your aim is to create an atmosphere of serenity, confidence and mutual trust. To maintain it requires that changes in position be gradual and

subtle. For example, if you are applying pressure and suddenly find that you are intolerably uncomfortable, begin to shift your position inch by inch to one more comfortable. You must know in advance which position you wish to assume and *gradually* move into it. Do not move while you are applying pressure. Instead, alternate movement with application of pressure. Press, then move a little; press, then move a little. Follow this procedure until the desired change of position is achieved. All movement and any alteration of position throughout the process of massage should combine grace with ease and subtlety in order not to disturb the receiver. For massage to work its magic, your every move must be magically imperceptible.

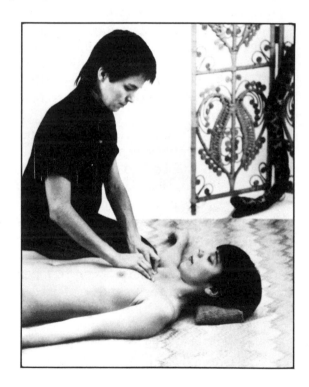

Keep your spine erect. Do not allow your back to sag. The upper back must be straight and relaxed, not hunched forward. The lower back must be as close to flat as possible. Avoid a concave depression in the small of the back, which results from the protrusion of the buttocks. As you massage, periodically check the orientation of your spine. If you are slouching or arched, straighten your spine slowly, but do not disturb the receiver.

Keep your shoulders loose and relaxed. Massaging with tense shoulders will cause much discomfort in a matter of minutes. To keep shoulders loose and relaxed is a little tricky at first, but practice will soon enable you to master that technique. Begin by letting your shoulders hang

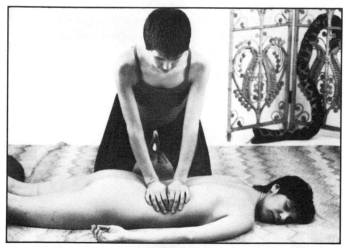

CORRECT

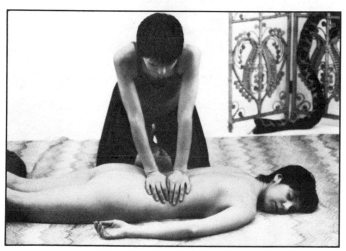

INCORRECT

loose. Concentrate, while you massage, on keeping your shoulders in this loose position. I don't mean by this that you should tense them in order to maintain their lowered position, but rather that you should concentrate on allowing them to hang low and loose. Focus on keeping your shoulders in this relaxed position as you work.

Do not use muscle power to apply pressure. When applying thumb pressure, use your body weight and your hara, not your shoulder muscle power. Imagine a magical force surging up from your torso, then streaming down your arms and into the receiver. Feel your strength rising up from within you. Do not rely on muscle power. Unless you are muscularly an extremely powerful person, you will soon exhaust your strength and tire. Try to develop your ability to massage from your hara. Hara is the Japanese word for the center of the energy of your body. The Japanese believe that when you function from your hara, all things are more easily accomplished, and I have certainly found this true in my own experience. Your hara is located one and a half inches below your navel.

Do not abuse your thumbs. Many of the pressure techniques require the use of your thumbs.

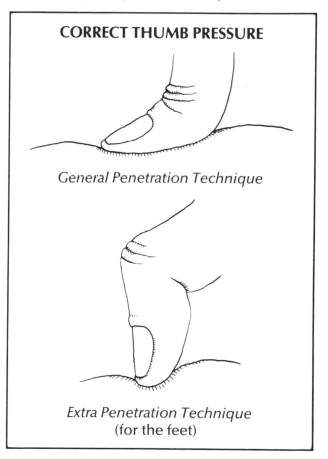

CORRECT THUMB PRESSURE

General Penetration Technique

Extra Penetration Technique
(for the feet)

If at any time you experience a shooting pain or a very tired sensation in your thumbs, switch to the use of your fingers, knuckles, elbows or knees. The heel of your foot and the heel of your hand are also useful tools.

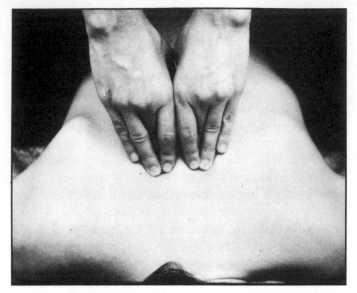

Your fingers can be used in much the same manner as your thumbs, because they, too, are soft and padded. Use your middle finger braced by the two fingers on either side of it. Remember to keep your shoulders loose and your spine erect as you work. There is a tendency to lose the correct posture when using a different technique.

When employing the knuckles, it is important to remember that much less pressure is required, because the knuckles, unlike the thumbs, are not well padded. Practice knuckle pressure on the re-

ceiver prior to beginning your first massage, so that you are aware of the extent of the receiver's tolerance for this technique. Knuckle pressure, like any other, is to be enjoyed and should not hurt. Keep a close watch on the receiver's face. The facial expressions will let you know whether the pressure you are applying is appropriate or not. If at any time you are uncertain about the amount of pressure, quietly ask your partner if it feels all right.

Elbows can be used with as much compassion and can be equally as effective as thumbs. Elbows are, however, very bony, so great care must be taken when you are using them in massage. If your frame is small and you are working on a

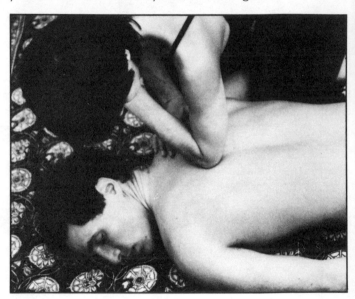

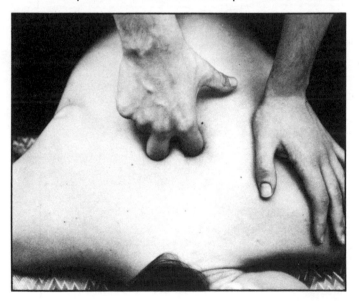

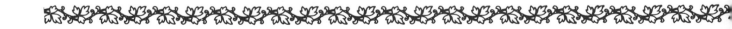

large person, your elbows can be especially useful along the spine. You will achieve excellent results with a minimal expenditure of effort and energy, and thereby conserve your strength for the rest of the massage. Apply pressure with your elbow to the tsubos, or pressure points, along one side of the spine, while resting the hand of your other arm on the receiver's back to provide a comforting touch. Repeat the same procedure for the other side.

Knees, too, can be useful tools. The knee can be applied to a specific pressure point and at the same time cover a general area. The most important thing to remember about this very sensitive addition to your repertoire of massage techniques is that the most prominent bony protrusion is the

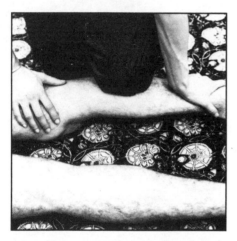

part of the knee that applies the pressure. Focus your attention on this protrusion as you work, so that you will know when you have applied enough pressure. Feel how deep it is penetrating. Only the bony protrusion is the tool. The rest of the knee is along for the ride.

The heels of your feet are useful in several instances. For example, if you're feeling a strain in your thumbs and the receiver's feet have yet to be massaged, use your feet. Walk on the bottom of your partner's feet. Apply pressure to the same areas as you would with your thumbs. Rest most of your body weight on each of the reflex points for three to five seconds. Some people can enjoy more pressure than others, so be sure to ask the receiver if the pressure is comfortable. You will

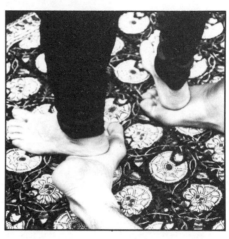

not be able to be quite as thorough working with your feet as with your thumbs, but you will be able to stimulate most of the reflex points. What you cannot reach with your feet can be completed afterwards with your thumbs or fingers. Maintain your balance with a chair if you feel you might fall. The heels can also be useful on the shoulders, the back of the legs and the buttocks. Always observe the receiver for reactions of pain.

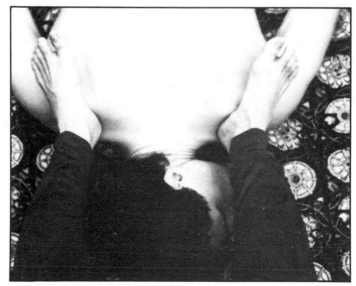

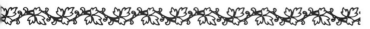

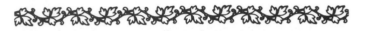

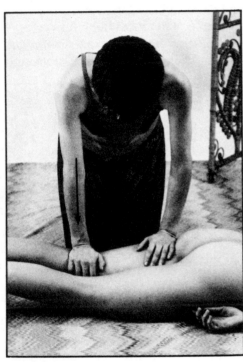

Positioning is important. Try to duplicate the positions illustrated in the text. These positions have been tested and proven to be comfortable and practical. Do not stretch to implement a technique. Do not work off balance.

The correct angle of penetration is important. Try as much as possible to apply pressure from directly above the area you are addressing. The angle of penetration should be perpendicular to the surface receiving the pressure. Your body weight will fall naturally onto the tsubo, and no muscle power will be needed.

The heel of your hand can be used for meridian tracing and specific point pressure. The entire surface of the heel of your hand is perfect for Technique #63, Upper Arm Lung Meridian Tracing. The bony protrusion at the wrist provides an

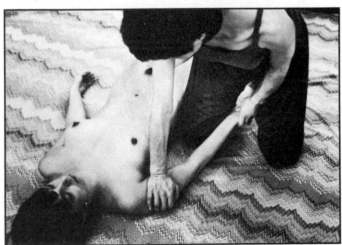

excellent tool for applying pressure to specific tsubos. Simply direct the force of the pressure down your arm, into this bony protrusion and into the receiver's body. Keep your hand relaxed as you work.

4)WHAT IS AN ECLECTIC MASSAGE?

The Random House College Dictionary definition of *eclectic* is: ''*Adj.* 1. selecting; choosing from various sources. 2. made up of what is selected from different sources. 3. not following any one system, as of philosophy, medicine, etc., but selecting and using what are considered the best elements of all systems . . . ''

Acupuncture Meridian Therapy without the use of a needle, which is also known as Acupressure, Acupuncture Holding/Pressure Point Therapy, Acu-therapy or Shiatsu, has been combined with Foot Reflexology, Touch for Health's Neurovascular Holding Points and Neuro-lymphatic Massage, Swedish Massage and many original techniques to produce an unusual system that integrates Eastern and Western approaches to body therapy. This book offers a new system of body maintenance and improvement, combining benefits from the most respected and effective disciplines in the field of physical health care. This system stimulates the body's own natural healing mechanism. Rather than directly effecting a cure, it encourages the body to do what it can to right a condition of ill health.

5)DISCIPLINES RELEVANT TO THIS SYSTEM OF ECLECTIC MASSAGE

The following pages highlight those aspects of the disciplines relevant to this system of eclectic massage that the author feels are most important for the reader's general knowledge. The information is by no means complete. For further information on any of the following disciplines, please refer to the Bibliography.

a)ACUPUNCTURE = *acu(s)/needle + punctura/puncture*

- A very thin needle penetrates the acupuncture points (tsubos), which are located along the meridians or energy pathway

- Penetration is shallow, no more than a few millimeters, and can be held for up to 30 minutes or longer

- Penetration executed efficiently results in little or no pain

- Meridians or energy pathways have been charted by modern electronic instruments

- Meridians are not only located on the surface of the body, as depicted in most drawings, but are also located deep within the body

- The meridian energy does not flow in a vessel, as does blood or lymph; therefore, the Western medical mind has had trouble accepting the ancient Eastern meridian theory, despite the fact that modern instruments have proven meridians do exist

- Many different theories attempt to explain how acupuncture works, but no one theory has found total acceptance

- It is important to remember that although Western medicine refuses to accept acupuncture into its mainstream, Eastern medicine continues to utilize acupuncture as a safe and effective method of anesthetizing patients during surgery. It also successfully treats many diseases and conditions with acupuncture

- Acupuncture relies on two basic methods for treating a health problem, the acupuncture of points close to the problem and the acupuncture of points distant from the problem

- The Western medical mind can more easily accept acupuncture of the *locus dolenti,* or points close to the problem, as a means of treatment, although acupuncture of distant points often proves more effective

- Acupuncture encourages the body's natural healing mechanism

- A total of fifty-nine meridians is commonly used in traditional Chinese acupuncture

- The twelve basic meridians and two other extra meridians, known as the governing and conception vessels, are the meridians of primary concern in this book

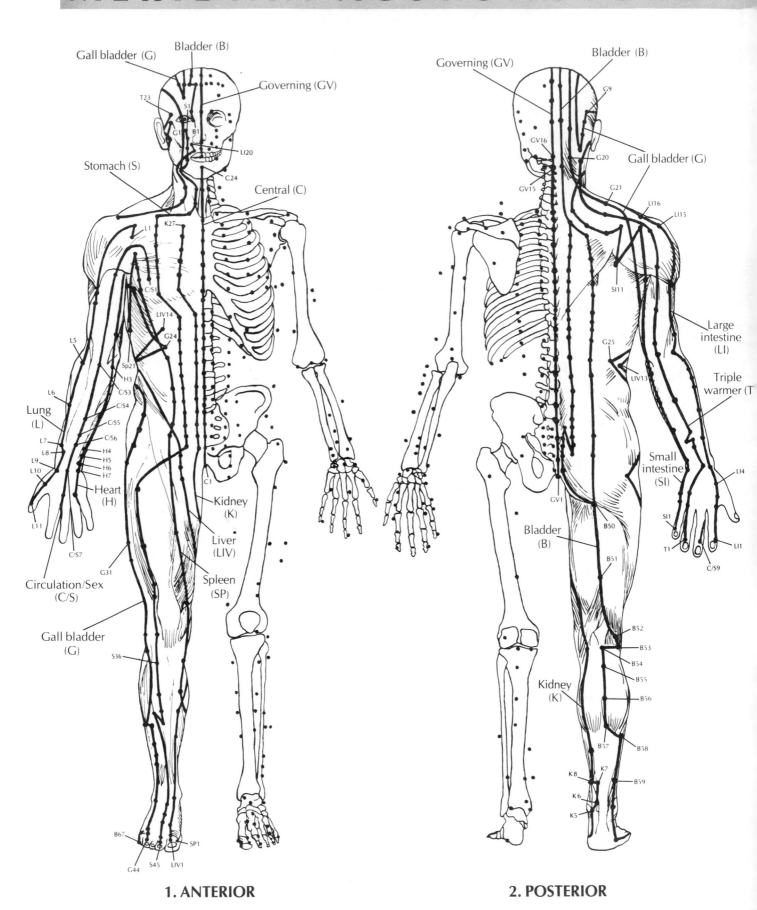

1. ANTERIOR

2. POSTERIOR

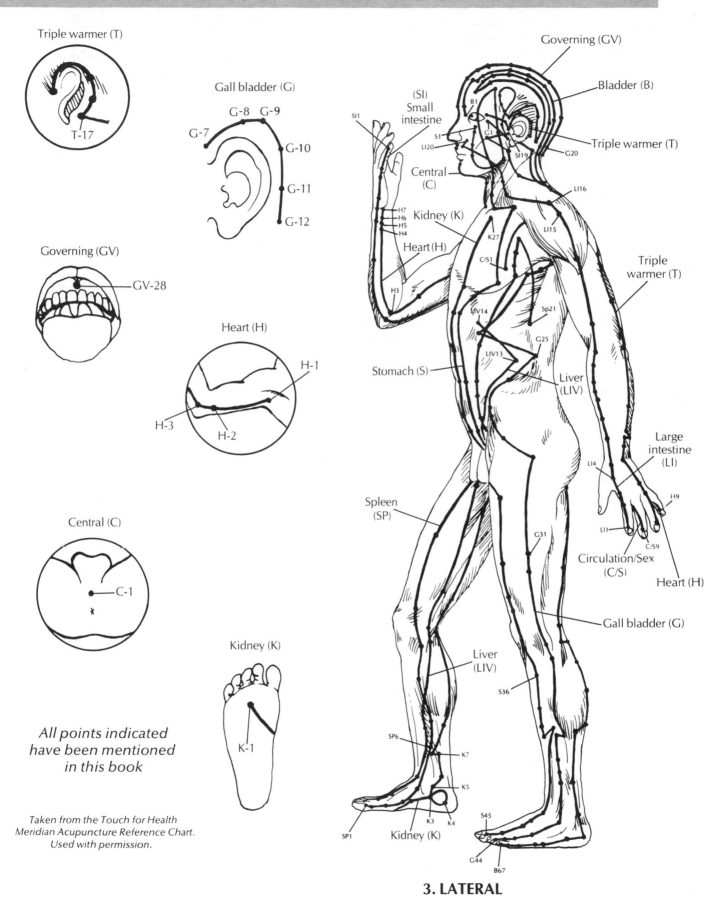

Triple warmer (T)

T-17

Gall bladder (G)

G-8 G-9

G-7

G-10

G-11

G-12

Governing (GV)

GV-28

Heart (H)

H-1

H-3

H-2

Central (C)

C-1

Kidney (K)

K-1

*All points indicated
have been mentioned
in this book*

Taken from the Touch for Health
Meridian Acupuncture Reference Chart.
Used with permission.

Governing (GV)

Bladder (B)

(SI)
Small
intestine

SI1

B1

G1

S1

LI20

SI19

Triple warmer (T)

G20

Central
(C)

LI16

Kidney (K)

H7
H6
H5
H4

K27

LI15

Heart (H)

C/S1

H3

Triple
warmer (T)

LIV14

Sp21

Stomach (S)

G25

Liver
(LIV)

LIV13

Large
intestine
(LI)

LI4

Spleen
(SP)

G31

LI1

C/S9

Circulation/Sex
(C/S)

H9

Heart (H)

Gall bladder (G)

Liver
(LIV)

S36

SP6

K7

K5

SP1

K3 K4

Kidney (K)

S45

G44

B67

3. LATERAL

MERIDIAN	**ASSOCIATED ORGAN OR AILMENT	ASSOCIATED MUSCLES
Conception/ Central	Brain	Supraspinatus
Governing	Spine & Nervous System	Teres Major
Stomach	Stomach tension & insomnia sinus & allergies headaches	Pectoralis Major Clavicular Levator Scapula Neck Muscles Brachioradialis
Spleen	Spleen Pancreas infections & fevers anemia	Latissimus Dorsi Trapezius Opponens Pollicis Triceps
Heart	Heart	Subscapularis
Small Intestine	Small Intestine digestive disturbances low back pain knee problems	Quadriceps Abdominals
Bladder	Bladder ankle problems & flat feet bunions emotional strain arthritis	Peroneus Sacrospinalis Tibialis
Kidney	Kidney skin problems dark marks under the eyes great thirst low back pain heart conditions eye & ear problems	Psoas Upper Trapezius Iliacus
Heart Constrictor/ Circulation-Sex	general circulation sex organs menstrual problems, breast pain, menopause prostate problems impotency sciatic pain bladder conditions	Gluteus Medius & Maximus Adductors Piriformis
Triple Heater/ Triple Warmer	Thyroid Adrenals Pancreas sugar problems infections	Teres Minor Sartorius Gracilis Soleus Gastrocnemius

MERIDIAN	**ASSOCIATED ORGAN OR AILMENT	ASSOCIATED MUSCLES
Gall Bladder	digestion & Gall Bladder conditions	Anterior Deltoid Popliteus
Liver	Liver grey spots interfering with vision glaucoma lengthy headaches	Pectoralis Major Sternal Rhomboids
Lungs	Lungs all lung conditions	Anterior Serratus Coracobrachialis Deltoids Diaphragm
Large Intestine	Large Intestine all conditions pertaining to the large intestines painful breasts and chest during menstruation restlessness & exhaustion headaches	Fascia Lata Hamstrings Quadratus Lumborum

**Associated Organ or Ailment. These ailments related to the associated organ, as well as many others not listed above, can be improved or cured by acupuncture meridian therapy.

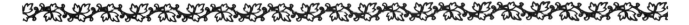

b) ACUPUNCTURE HOLDING/ PRESSURE POINTS

(Acupressure or Acu-therapy: Misnomers, because *acu-* means needle, and no needles are used.)

- No needles are used in acupuncture holding/ pressure points

- Light finger contact is applied to the skin at the acupuncture points or tsubos for holding points and heavy pressure for pressure points

- As with acupuncture, repeated applications of the light or heavy finger contact are usually necessary to effect a cure or lessen symptoms

- The great advantage of acupuncture holding/ pressure points is that you can help yourself

- Some doctors and chiropractors are now teaching their patients the acupuncture holding/pressure points relevant to the patient's particular condition

- Holding points must be held for 20-30 seconds in order to elicit a reaction

- Touch for Health utilizes acupuncture holding points

- Shiatsu utilizes acupuncture pressure points

- Pressure points must be held for 3-10 seconds or up to one minute depending upon the severity of the condition

c) SHIATSU =
shi/fingers + atsu/pressure

- This discipline primarily utilizes thumb pressure which is applied to the tsubos

- Most shiatsu is based on the twelve basic and two extra ancient Chinese acupuncture meridians discussed above under ACUPUNCTURE, although some practitioners use other meridian systems as well

- The Japanese Ministry of Health and Welfare states that Shiatsu therapy can "correct internal malfunctioning, promote health, and treat specific diseases"

- Shiatsu pressure is firmer than the light contact used for acupuncture holding points

- Pressure is generally held for three to ten seconds or one minute depending upon the severity of the condition

- Chronic and acute conditions usually require repeated applications of pressure to effect an improvement; however, under certain circumstances immediate results are noted after one application

- Shiatsu treatment need not be a painful experience, although occasional discomfort is sometimes inevitable

- Shiatsu evolved from ancient Chinese techniques of massage and manipulation in the early part of this century

- Each point along a meridian corresponds to and helps effect a change in a particular organ or part of the body

- Shiatsu encourages the body's natural healing mechanism to function optimally

- Shiatsu is administered slowly, quietly and with great compassion

d) REFLEXOLOGY *Hand & Foot*

- The body is divided into ten different zones which extend into the feet and the hands *See page 44*

- Each area of the foot corresponds to a specific organ or part of the body

- Nerves that pass through the body's organs and muscles terminate in the hands and feet

- Applying pressure to a particular area of the foot or hand stimulates the flow of energy, blood, nutrients and nerve impulses to its corresponding zone of the body

- Crystalline deposits of uric acid and calcium that form at the nerve endings prevent the nerve from functioning at its peak efficiency

- Pressure applied to the reflex points disintegrates crystalline deposits on the nerve endings. it also affects the entire nerve as well as those muscles and organs it innervates

- Once crushed, crystalline deposits can be reabsorbed into the bloodstream and excreted in the urine

- Reflexology stimulates the body's own natural healing mechanism

- A firm pressure is required, but the object is NOT to inflict pain

- Two or three applications of pressure daily are required to effect a change in a condition

- There are many different schools of reflexology, each with its own interpretation of where the reflex points are located

- All schools agree, however, that the precise locations of the nerve endings vary slightly in each individual

- The following charts take into consideration many different schools, plus some of the author's own discoveries *See page 43 and 67*

HAND REFLEXOLOGY

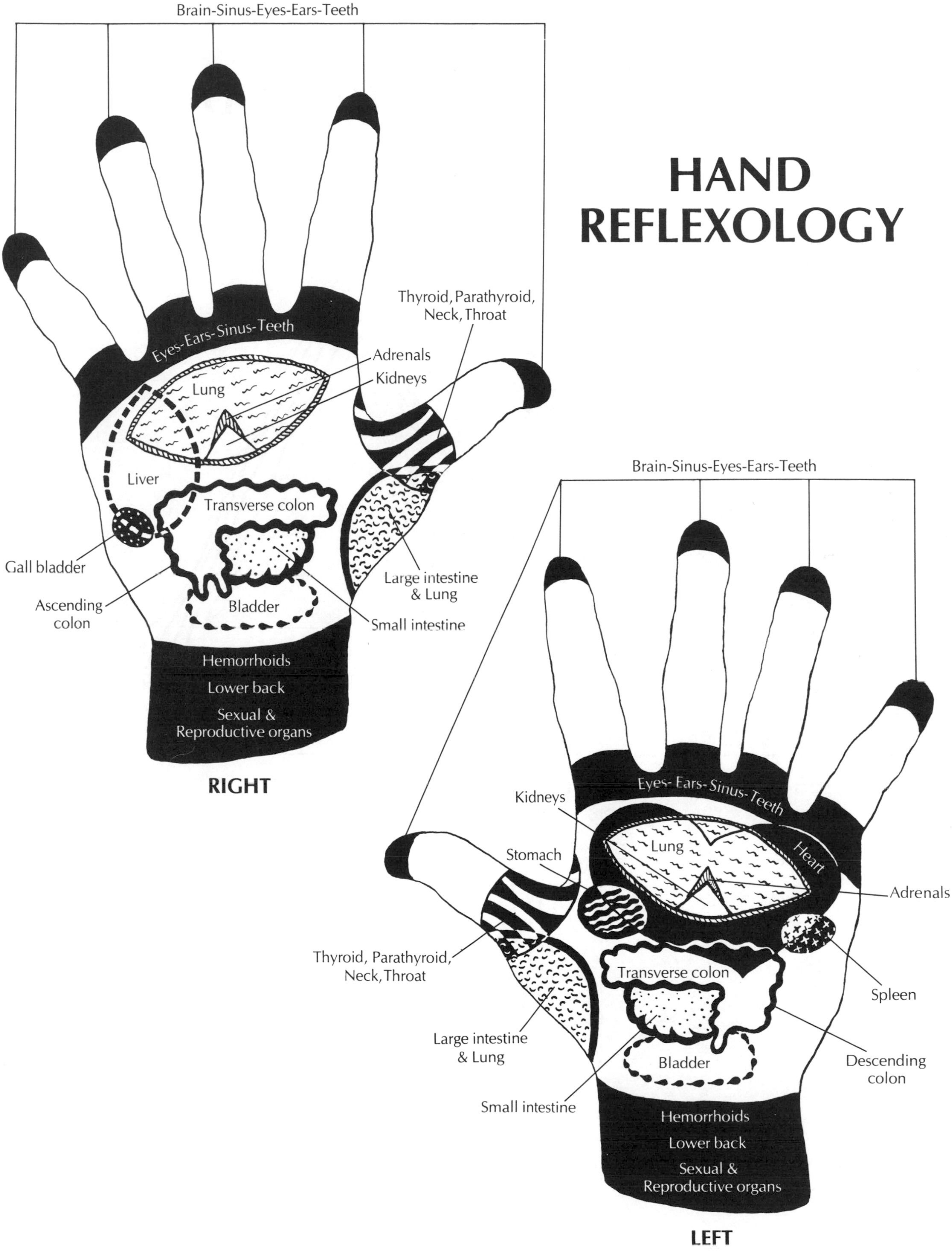

Brain-Sinus-Eyes-Ears-Teeth

Eyes-Ears-Sinus-Teeth

Thyroid, Parathyroid, Neck, Throat

Adrenals
Kidneys

Lung

Liver

Transverse colon

Gall bladder

Ascending colon

Bladder

Large intestine & Lung

Small intestine

Hemorrhoids
Lower back
Sexual & Reproductive organs

RIGHT

Brain-Sinus-Eyes-Ears-Teeth

Eyes-Ears-Sinus-Teeth

Kidneys

Stomach

Lung

Heart

Adrenals

Transverse colon

Spleen

Thyroid, Parathyroid, Neck, Throat

Large intestine & Lung

Bladder

Descending colon

Small intestine

Hemorrhoids
Lower back
Sexual & Reproductive organs

LEFT

ZONES OF THE BODY

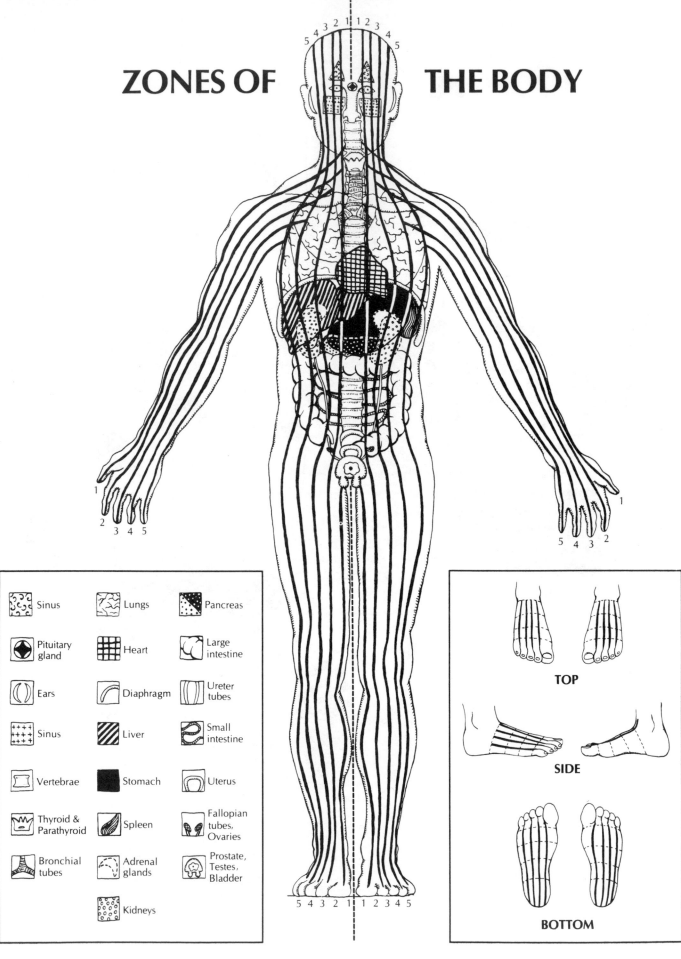

Sinus

Pituitary gland

Ears

Sinus

Vertebrae

Thyroid & Parathyroid

Bronchial tubes

Kidneys

Lungs

Heart

Diaphragm

Liver

Stomach

Spleen

Adrenal glands

Pancreas

Large intestine

Ureter tubes

Small intestine

Uterus

Fallopian tubes, Ovaries

Prostate, Testes, Bladder

TOP

SIDE

BOTTOM

e) TOUCH FOR HEALTH

Touch for Health utilizes the techniques of Applied Kinesiology to encourage the body's natural healing mechanism. Applied Kinesiology has derived some of its methods from Oriental Medicine. Some of the methods used to achieve results are:

1) *Muscle Testing*

2) *Neuro-vascular Holding Points*

3) *Neuro-lymphatic Massage Points*

4) *Meridian Tracing*

1) MUSCLE TESTING

- Applied Kinesiology is a science that has proven each muscle to be affected by the function of a particular organ(s)

- Muscle testing is the method used to determine if a muscle is strong or weak

- Muscle testing indicates the ability or inability of a muscle and its associated organ to function at peak energy efficiency

- Applied Kinesiology utilizes neuro-vascular holding points, neuro-lymphatic massage, meridian therapy, origin and insertion massage (simultaneously massaging the origin and insertion of a muscle), exercise and other methods to restore the proper function to the muscle and its related organ

- Applied Kinesiology is used extensively by chiropractors and the layperson's adaptation of it is taught by certified Touch for Health instructors

2) NEURO-VASCULAR HOLDING POINTS

- Neuro-vascular holding points or receptors were discovered in the 1930's by Dr. Terence Bennett

- George Goodheart, D.C., revealed the relationship between the neuro-vascular holding points and the musculoskeletal system

The neuro-vascular receptors, when blocked, will prevent the occurrence of the lactic acid response, which occurs naturally each time a muscle contracts

- Connect with the neuro-vascular holding points by applying a light finger-pad contact

- Feel for a light pulse not directly related to the heartbeat. If the pulse is difficult to locate, gently stretch the skin and the pulse will become noticeable

- This pulsation is thought to be a result of the capillary beds' microscopic throbbing

- Hold the receptors until the pulses become synchronized. This usually occurs within twenty seconds, although five, ten or more minutes may be necessary

- Neuro-vascular holding points are believed to improve the capillary circulation of blood to the muscle and its related organ

- Most of the neuro-vascular holding points are situated on the skull *See pages 152 & 153*

3) NEURO-LYMPHATIC MASSAGE POINTS

- Dr. Frank Chapman was the first to discover neuro-lymphatic massage points or receptors

- George Goodheart, D.C., systematically correlated each neuro-lymphatic receptor to one or more muscles

- When a neuro-lymphatic receptor is blocked, its correspondent muscles are unable to function normally

- Massage the neuro-lymphatics by applying a medium-firm pressure with your thumbs or fingers

- Those neuro-lymphatics that are tender are most in need of massage

- Use a clockwise massaging motion. If the tenderness does not disappear within fifteen to thirty seconds, switch to a counter-clockwise massaging motion

SCHEMATIC
THE LYMPHATIC DRAINAGE SYSTEM

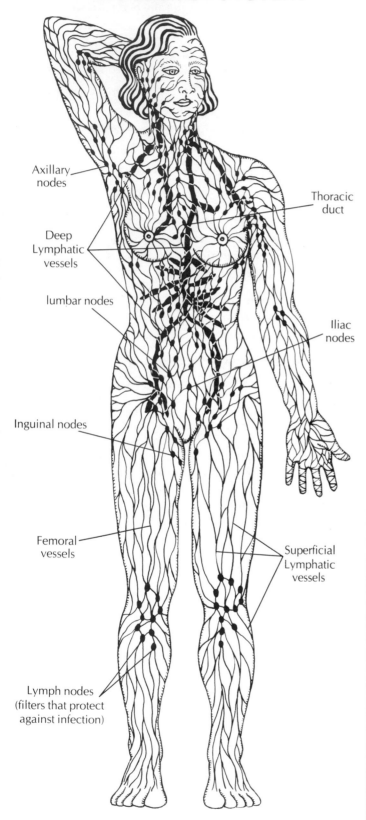

Axillary nodes

Deep Lymphatic vessels

lumbar nodes

Inguinal nodes

Femoral vessels

Lymph nodes (filters that protect against infection)

Thoracic duct

Iliac nodes

Superficial Lymphatic vessels

ANTERIOR

Lymph vessels return excess tissue fluid and cellular waste products to the blood stream.

NEURO-LYMPHATIC MASSAGE POINTS

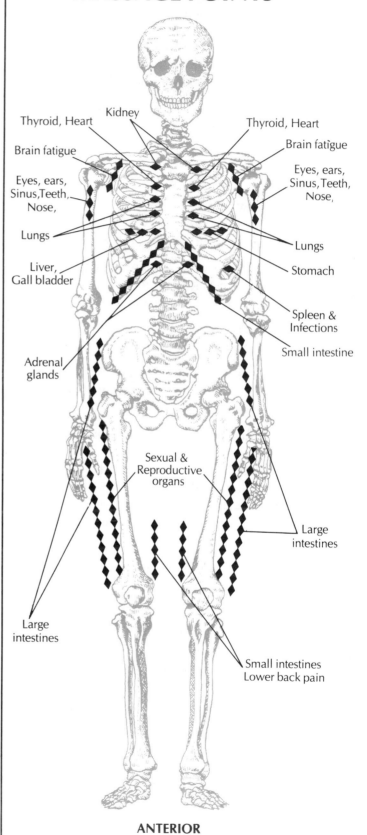

Thyroid, Heart

Kidney

Thyroid, Heart

Brain fatigue

Brain fatigue

Eyes, ears, Sinus,Teeth, Nose,

Eyes, ears, Sinus,Teeth, Nose,

Lungs

Lungs

Liver, Gall bladder

Stomach

Spleen & Infections

Small intestine

Adrenal glands

Sexual & Reproductive organs

Large intestines

Large intestines

Small intestines Lower back pain

ANTERIOR

- The neuro-lymphatics generally become less tender as you massage them, for release of the backed-up lymphatic system is being achieved

- Most of the neuro-lymphatics are located on the torso (front and back), although some are located on the legs and arms

- If the neuro-lymphatic tenderness still exists after fifteen or thirty seconds of first clockwise and then counter-clockwise massaging, the muscle and organ associated with the particular neuro-lymphatic will require many more applications over a period of time in order for the blockage to be released

- The neuro-lymphatic massage points or receptors flush the body's lymph system.

- When a body is overloaded with toxins, the lymphatic receptors become tender or painful to the touch, and act as an alarm system

- Some of the neuro-lymphatic massage points correspond to the location of the lymph glands or nodules; however, many do not directly relate in a physical sense

- The lymph is also responsible for the transport of fats, hormones and proteins as well as for the production of antibodies

4) MERIDIAN TRACING

- Lightly trace or follow the line or course of a meridian several times from its origin to its termination

- If tracing a meridian from its origin to its point of termination makes the receiver feel uneasy, try reversing the flow of the meridian several times or alternating its flow from origin to termination and then from termination to origin a few times. This is known as flushing a meridian. Complete the procedure by tracing the meridian several times in the correct direction. This procedure will often correct the flow of a meridian that is reversed *Refer to pages 38 & 39 for the exact location of the meridians for tracing purposes.*

f) SWEDISH MASSAGE

- Swedish massage improves blood and lymph circulation

- It breaks down adhesions, reduces swelling and encourages wounds to heal

- It improves the flexibility of joints and increases their range of motion

- When using effleurage on the limbs, always begin at the extremity and continue upward toward the heart in order to return stagnant blood back to the heart for recirculation

- Swedish massage uses more vigorous and stimulating techniques than Shiatsu

- There are five basic massage techniques:

  1) Effleurage—a long stroking motion, deep or superficial, in the direction of the heart, to improve circulation and lymph flow throughout the body as well as to improve nutrition and functioning of muscles

  2) Petrissage—the kneading, picking up, squeezing and rolling of the muscles to stimulate the deep blood and lymph vessels and to strengthen the muscles

  3) Friction—a penetrating circular movement, applied primarily to the joints, to effect destruction of adhesions

  4) Vibration— of the forearm, hand and fingers to stimulate the nervous system

  5) Tapotment—a chopping, slapping, hacking, beating, cupping motion, implemented with the hands open or closed, to stimulate the muscles — Tapotment can also either sedate or stimulate the nerves, depending upon the duration and intensity of its application

- Swedish massage does not, for the most part, claim to affect or assist directly the functioning of internal organs. Nor does it concern itself with the movement of energy or the meridian system and its pressure points

THE BLOOD CIRCULATORY SYSTEM
SCHEMATIC

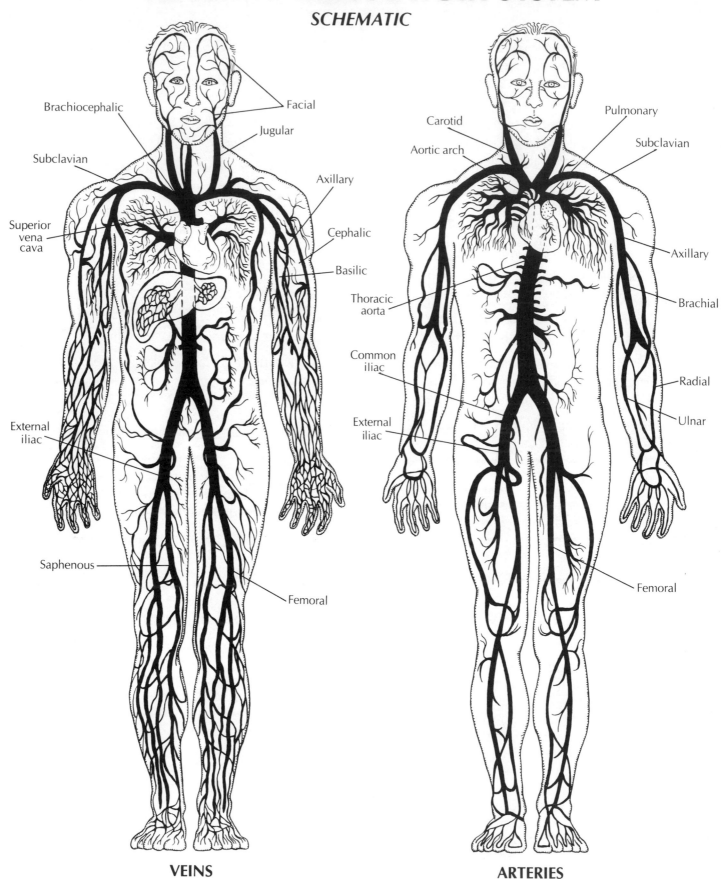

Brachiocephalic

Facial

Jugular

Subclavian

Axillary

Superior vena cava

Cephalic

Basilic

External iliac

Saphenous

Femoral

Carotid

Pulmonary

Aortic arch

Subclavian

Axillary

Thoracic aorta

Brachial

Common iliac

Radial

External iliac

Ulnar

Femoral

VEINS

Veins transport deoxygenated blood to the heart and lungs for recirculation.

ARTERIES

Arteries transport oxygenated blood away from the heart to all parts of the body.

6)BASIC SKELETAL & MUSCULAR ANATOMY

- Bones fall into four categories: long, short, flat and irregular

- All bones have a porous inner portion and an outer covering of hard, compact bone

- Bones provide support and protection as well as making movement possible in coordination with the muscular system

- Bones are found in pairs, one on each side of the body

- Bones store calcium and form red blood cells

- Nutrient rich blood and lymph fluids move into and out of bone tissue

ANATOMY OF A LONG BONE

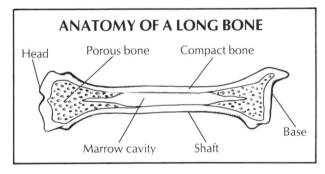

Head   Porous bone   Compact bone

Marrow cavity   Shaft   Base

The following skeletal charts will give you a good sense of the bony structure or foundation that provides places of attachment for all the muscles, so that you will not harm the receiver while implementing pressure points. Have someone lie down on the floor. Try to visualize where the bones are located in the person's body. If you cannot quite determine a bone's location, feel for it while making frequent visual checks to the following charts.

- Muscles consist of fibers or cells, which, if contracted, pull bones and effect movement of the body

- Muscles are found in pairs, one on each side of the body

- All muscles have two ends, an origin and an insertion, which attach or connect to bones, ligaments or cartilage

- The origin of a muscle is usually closer to the center of your body

- The belly of a muscle is the fullest or broadest part of a muscle

- Massaging the origin and insertion of a muscle in unison helps to strengthen that muscle

- You can relax a muscle by feathering, by a light gliding motion or by a medium-pressure pulling motion. When implementing any of these techniques, work from the belly of the muscle toward the origin and insertion in order to relieve muscle cramps or spasms

- The same feathering and pulling motions, when utilized from the origin and insertion toward the belly of the muscle, will strengthen a weak muscle

- Muscles store physical and emotional trauma which form a knot or hard spot. Such traumatized areas are usually swollen to some degree and hotter than healthy, normal tissue and are also known as adhesions or energy blockages

ANATOMY OF A MUSCLE

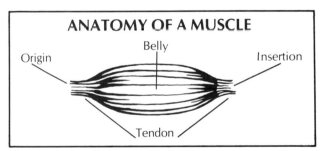

Belly

Origin   Insertion

Tendon

The following muscle charts must be reviewed before beginning your first massage. It is helpful to the beginner to have an understanding and mental image of the major muscles of the body. Remember, you are not massaging or applying pressure to the skin, but to the muscles and the core of the body. A deep, penetrating massage or pressure need not be painful. An understanding of the muscular system will allow you to handle the body skillfully and with great compassion.

THE SKELETAL SYSTEM

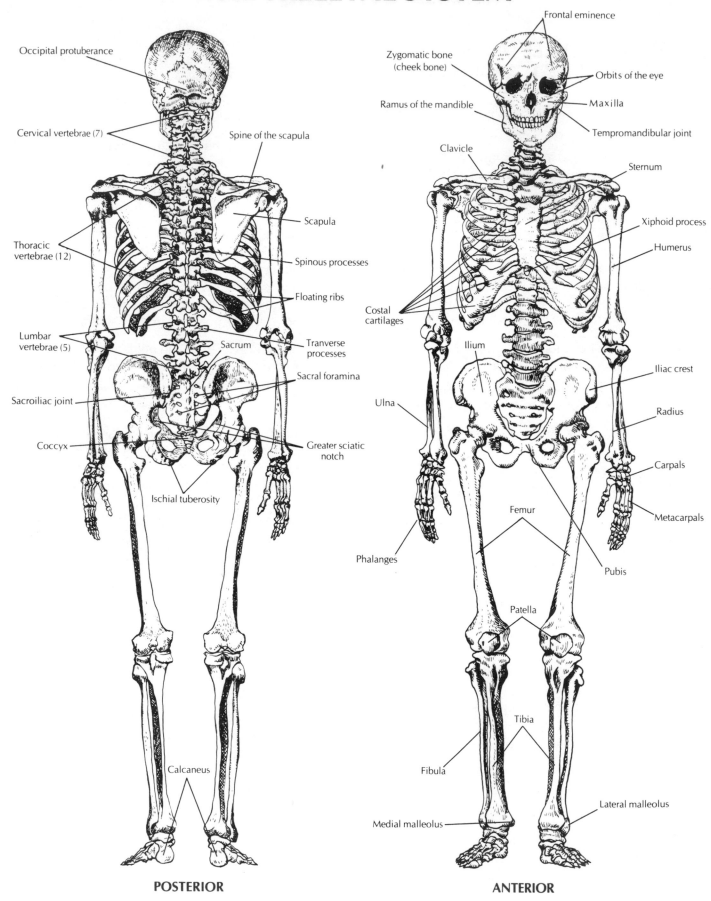

Occipital protuberance

Cervical vertebrae (7)

Spine of the scapula

Scapula

Thoracic vertebrae (12)

Spinous processes

Floating ribs

Lumbar vertebrae (5)

Sacrum

Tranverse processes

Sacral foramina

Sacroiliac joint

Coccyx

Greater sciatic notch

Ischial tuberosity

Calcaneus

Frontal eminence

Zygomatic bone (cheek bone)

Orbits of the eye

Ramus of the mandible

Maxilla

Tempromandibular joint

Clavicle

Sternum

Xiphoid process

Humerus

Costal cartilages

Ilium

Iliac crest

Ulna

Radius

Carpals

Metacarpals

Femur

Phalanges

Pubis

Patella

Tibia

Fibula

Lateral malleolus

Medial malleolus

POSTERIOR

ANTERIOR

50

THE MUSCULAR SYSTEM

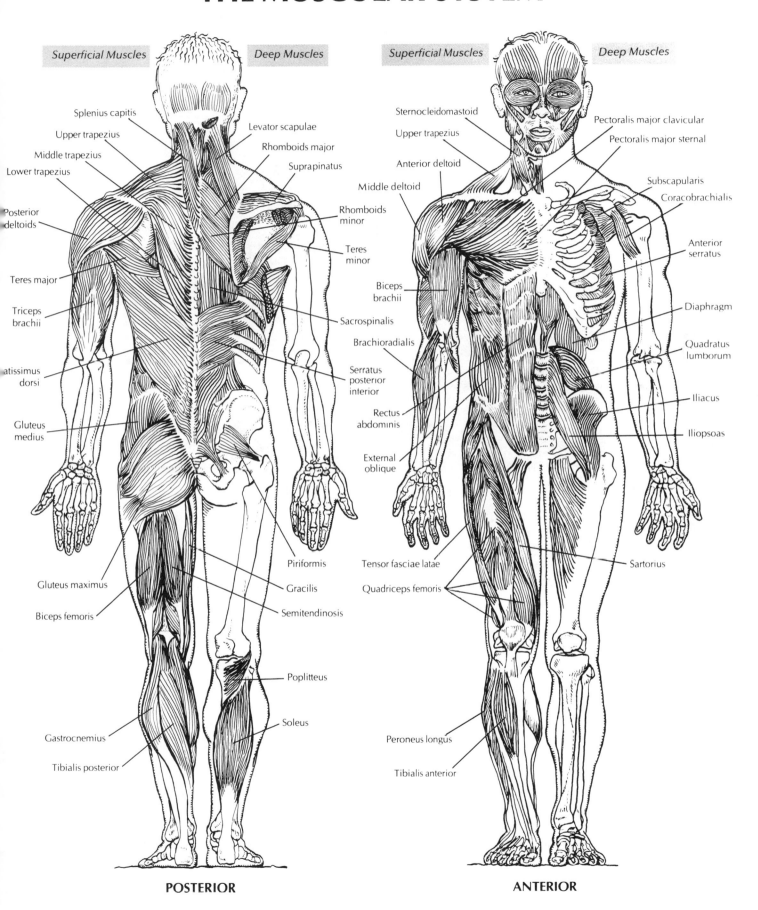

POSTERIOR

ANTERIOR

Superficial Muscles — Deep Muscles

Splenius capitis
Upper trapezius
Middle trapezius
Lower trapezius
Posterior deltoids
Teres major
Triceps brachii
Latissimus dorsi
Gluteus medius
Gluteus maximus
Biceps femoris
Gastrocnemius
Tibialis posterior

Levator scapulae
Rhomboids major
Suprapinatus
Rhomboids minor
Teres minor
Sacrospinalis
Serratus posterior interior
Piriformis
Gracilis
Semitendinosis
Poplitteus
Soleus

Superficial Muscles — Deep Muscles

Sternocleidomastoid
Upper trapezius
Anterior deltoid
Middle deltoid
Biceps brachii
Brachioradialis
Rectus abdominis
External oblique
Tensor fasciae latae
Quadriceps femoris
Peroneus longus
Tibialis anterior

Pectoralis major clavicular
Pectoralis major sternal
Subscapularis
Coracobrachialis
Anterior serratus
Diaphragm
Quadratus lumborum
Iliacus
Iliopsoas
Sartorius

CHAPTER IV

How to Give A Complete 60-Minute Body Massage

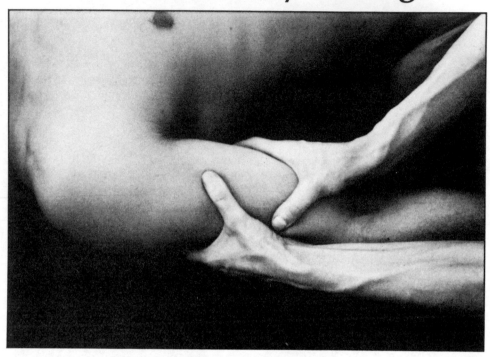

INTRODUCTION

The Complete 60-Minute Body Massage is intended for use by couples or friends who would like to exchange massages on a regular weekly basis. Partners should read this section together and practice each technique prior to the first massage, not only to gain knowledge of each of the procedures but also to share the actual physical experience of each technique. Consequently, the receiver will relax more easily and the doer will feel more self-confident. The massage, in turn, will be a more rewarding exchange. This introduction is written primarily for the doer, although some mention is made of the receiver's responsibility.

Responsibility and commitment to the massage are essential components of its success. Both the doer and the receiver must be prepared to fulfill their responsibilities in order to assure a pleasurable exchange.

As the receiver, you must make every effort to relax. You should breathe slowly and take deeper breaths when a pressure point is tender or painful. Your deep inhalation will alert the doer to reduce the force of the pressure being applied. Words are usually unnecessary, but if the deep breathing method fails to alert the doer to your discomfort, verbally express your malaise and request that less pressure be applied. Don't hide the pain you feel. Avoid talking as much as possible. Speak only when it is absolutely necessary, and let the magic of massage flow from the doer's hands into your body. Keep your eyes closed. Allow your mind to free-associate. Don't focus on your thoughts, but simply let them pass or wander through your mind. As the receiver, it is your responsibility NOT to help the doer by lifting your arms, legs or head. Since the doer is usually strong enough to lift your appendages, your help is unnecessary. Finally, if you, as the receiver, find yourself falling asleep, don't fight it, surrender completely and let go.

It is the doer's responsibility to be calm, compassionate and in control, for otherwise the receiver will not feel secure enough to let go. Perform techniques slowly. Quick or vigorous massaging is not conducive to the calm you wish to achieve and prevents the receiver's body from achieving deep relaxation. Whenever you utilize kneading techniques, perform them slowly without the use of oils.

Improved blood and lymphatic circulation can also be effected through slowly executed massage and pressure techniques. Your aim is to sedate, not stimulate, the receiver. As life offers more than enough stimulation, massage, in my opinion, should be sedating in order to provide maximum benefits. Once the body has been successfully relaxed, so that energy blockages as well as muscle tension can be released, the lymph and blood circulation will automatically improve. Sedation of the receiver's mind and body is the most effective way to release stored tension on both the emotional and physical levels.

It is also the doer's responsibility to remind the receiver to breathe. The reminder can be verbal, or you can exaggerate your inhaling and exhaling until the receiver gets the message. Most people hold their breath without knowing it. If you allow the receiver to do so frequently throughout a massage, the results will be less releasing and less relaxing.

Avoid losing contact with the receiver's body whenever you change techniques or switch positions. Always keep one hand or some part of your body in contact with the receiver's body. If you do not, the receiver will usually experience a mild shock due to the unexpected withdrawal. The eyes will suddenly open and the receiver will often sit up with a start and wonder if something is wrong. When it is absolutely necessary that you remove yourself entirely from the receiver's body, your departure and your return to contact must be very gradual, so that the receiver doesn't experience a feeling of separation. Generally, it is far simpler to remain in constant contact with the receiver's body.

Occasionally the receiver may say, "Oh, that feels good!" or "Could you do more of that technique?" You, as the doer should always acknowledge such comments. Tell the receiver that you will remain with the technique a little longer than usual and that you will return to it later during the massage. A receiver's compliment to you on a particular technique usually indicates the fulfillment of a great physical or emotional need. Often the receiver will sigh deeply rather than speak. A deep sigh also signals your duty to spend a little more time on the technique. Do not deny the receiver. The extra attention you give to a particular need communicates your understanding, your sensitivity and your willingness to help the receiver. It will also significantly increase the benefits of the particular technique.

There are three basic degrees of pressure: light, medium and heavy. No set standard exists for any of these three degrees, as each person is capable of enjoying and tolerating different amounts of pressure and pain. Learn your receiver's tolerance level and observe the face for indications of pain or pleasure. Remember, too, that firm pressure is not always applied with the same amount of force, even when massaging the same receiver. For example, firm pressure applied to the eyes will obviously differ in force from firm pressure applied to the arms or legs. The part of the body being massaged or receiving pressure determines how much force you apply. It is extremely difficult to describe the application of pressure without becoming slightly esoteric. The application of heavy pressure without causing the receiver pain is esssential to the successful practice of massage. Even some professional massage therapists do not know how to apply pressure correctly, so don't be to discouraged if you fail to grasp the method of application immediately.

Pressure applied incorrectly results in a brutal, insensitive massage. The pressure you apply must be the end-result of a magical force hidden deep within you and rising up from your hara, then following down your arms and into the receiver's body. Hara, remember, is the Japanese word for the center of the energy of your body and is located approximately one-and-a-half inches below your navel. Here resides the strength and the sensitivity needed to accomplish a successful, compassionate and magical massage.

The Japanese believe that when you function from the hara, you can achieve what would normally be difficult or impossible. Hara, in Western terms, can most easily be described as functioning from your gut or relying on your instincts. You've heard of "gut reaction." Gut reactions are almost always correct or accurate. For example, imagine you are with someone when they receive shocking news over the telephone. Your gut reaction or instincts tell you to hold or console the person. Or imagine you are walking down the street and coming toward you is someone who looks like trouble. Chances are, your instincts will tell you to cross the street to avoid the trouble. By the same token, if you apply pressure or massage from your hara, you will instinctively know how much pressure to apply. Do not consciously try to determine how much pressure to apply. Let your instincts or gut reaction be your guide. Remember, don't use muscle power. Pain is not your objective. Use hara or gut force. Excellent results can be achieved with less pressure and a minimum of pain.

There are several different types of pain. It is important to be aware of the type with which you are dealing as you massage. Always apply pressure slowly, and take the time to notice the receiver's reaction in order to reduce the possibility of inflicting pain.

1) "Tender" means that the pressure applied hurts a little, but not enough to be painful.

2) "Good pain" hurts, but the receiver knows or can feel that the pressure is helping and therefore, the pain is worth tolerating.

3) "Bad pain" is usually the result of too much pressure, of a slip of the hand or thumb, or of pressure beyond the receiver's tolerance threshold.

Whenever you apply pressure that causes pain, the doer should be sure to "make nice" afterwards. Making nice indicates to the receiver that you are aware of the discomfort. It is also a perfect way to say, "I'm sorry." Make nice by giving a few light circular massages to the painful area or by gently holding the spot with your thumb, fingers or entire hand.

It is important to apply pressure slowly so that you can determine the shape of the bony structures under the skin. When you're certain of the form the bone assumes beneath a particular pressure point, you are less likely to slip and harm the receiver. When applying pressure to the limbs, each application should slightly "roll" or move the limb. If it doesn't, chances are that you are applying too much force behind your pressure or that the receiver is tense. Your aim is not to nail the limb to the floor. Again, remember to draw upon the force within your hara.

If the receiver has a diagnosed condition for the points you are utilizing, repeat the technique to increase the benefits. For example, by applying repeated pressure to the points that correspond to the liver, gall bladder, stomach, heart, spleen, lungs, eyes or ears, you can encourage the body's natural healing mechanism to take over and help to correct the condition.

Diseases or illnesses are either acute or chronic. Acute illnesses or conditions occur suddenly, and the symptoms are usually quite severe. Chronic illnesses have a long duration, sometimes months and often years, and are conditions that recur frequently. Whether chronic or acute, most illnesses respond well to frequently repeated applications of pressure or massage. The more frequently the organs' corresponding points are contacted, the greater the results. Contacting these points several times daily will, over a period of time, speed the recovery of both acute and chronic conditions.

Don't get discouraged. Keep at it. As most conditions take years to evolve, you can't expect to improve or cure them overnight. Rarely will you notice immediate results. Weeks or months are usually needed in order to effect a significantly noticeable difference. Some improvement is, however, usually apparent after one or two weeks of frequent daily applications. Patience will reward you.

The Complete 60-Minute Body Massage is a synthesis of Acupuncture pressure points, Shiatsu, Touch for Health, Foot Reflexology, Swedish Massage and original techniques. The meridians, acupuncture points, neuro-lymphatic drainage points, reflex points and Swedish techniques illustrated in this chapter were briefly discussed in Chapter III, Section 5.

The muscles and bones mentioned in this section are diagrammed in Chapter III, Section 6. Review the drawings before attempting to give your first massage. This basic anatomical information is essential to your success.

This section of *The Magic of Massage* occasionally mentions a relationship between a particular organ and muscle. Applied Kinesiology, discussed in Section 5e of Chapter III, has proven that specific muscles relate to particular organs. Whenever the text states that a particular muscle is related to a specific organ, the information has been derived from the science of Applied Chiropractic Kinesiological Diagnosis and Technique.

Feathering, utilized only once, in Technique #30 for Feathering the Spine, can also be used as a farewell to the part of the body you have been massaging and as a greeting to the part of the body you are about to massage. Feathering is done with the finger tips. Your aim is to create the sensation of a feather lightly gliding over the receiver's body. Maintain a very light contact with your finger tips while gliding them over the skin. Feathering can be done in any direction. Its light, gliding motion signals the brain to relax the area being feathered and thereby prepares it for massage or suggests a farewell. Feathering can be utilized before and after many of the techniques discussed in The Complete 60-Minute Body Massage. This feather in the margin or between techniques indicates an appropriate time to feather. The use of feathering is optional and is not included in the total time calculations. It is, however, a delightful addition to any massage.

The Complete 60-Minute Body Massage is presented in the following format:

NAME OF THE TECHNIQUE

Purpose: Why you do the technique and what organs, muscles or part of the body is affected.
Positioning: What position is most practical to assume. If this position is not comfortable for your particular body type, improvise until you find one that is.
Procedure: How to execute the technique, along with important tips to remember while implementing it.
Repetition: How many times the technique should be repeated during the massage.
Time: Approximately how much time is required to complete the technique. The time allotted cannot be very exacting, because each individual will require repetition of the techniques for the particular conditions that are troublesome to them. Obviously, someone who is very ill or run-down will require more repetitions than someone who is in reasonably good health.

Remember that in the magic of massage, fifty percent of the success is determined by the quality of your touch and fifty percent by your desire to help. Technique and know-how are important, but only as vehicles for your touch and your desire to help.

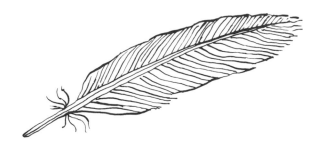

THE BACK

It is advisable to begin a massage with the back because many people experience a stiffening of the neck when lying in a prone position. The receiver must, after all, lie prone with the head turned to one side for the ten or fifteen minutes required by the doer to massage and apply pressure to the back. When you end a massage with the back, the receiver will often sit up, rotate the neck and try to massage it. Of course, the doer can, at this point, massage away the stiffness in the receiver's shoulders and tension in the neck, but it is psychologically unwise to conclude a session in this manner. Indeed, it's ridiculous to ruin one hour of wonderful manipulation by leaving the receiver with a pain in the neck. Therefore, unless you are sure the receiver will not develop a stiff neck, begin the massage with the back and follow the sequence of techniques listed below. Use slow, calm massaging motions and cautious, but firm applications of pressure to specific points.

All techniques should be executed quietly, slowly and with great compassion. There are two very important rules that must be remembered. One is NEVER to apply pressure directly over the spinous processes. The other is NEVER to apply

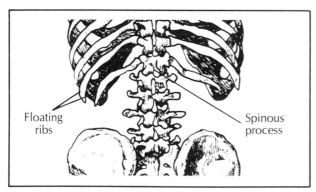

Floating ribs

Spinous process

too much open-handed pressure to the lower back, for there are no ribs in the lower back to absorb such pressure. Also, it is important that heavy pressure NOT be applied over the last two floating ribs as they can break quite easily.

For the sake of clarity some of the photographs do not show a pillow under the receiver's legs.

1) THE FIRST TOUCH

Purpose: The First Touch is a subtle way of letting the receiver know you are ready to begin. Words are unnecessary.

Positioning: Sit, Japanese style, parallel to the receiver between the body and the arm.

Procedure: The First Touch is executed with the side of your leg, not with your hands. Position yourself next to the receiver, but do not make contact at this time. The side of your body should be approximately 1-1½ inches from the receiver's body. Remain perfectly still for 10-15 seconds. Try to release everyday thoughts from your mind. To aid you, take a few breaths. When you are ready to begin, gently shift your body weight until your leg comes in contact with the side of the receiver's body. You have now completed the First Touch.

Repetition: Repetition of this technique is necessary only if you are interrupted and must start again.

Time: Allow 15 seconds to relax prior to making your first touch. When both you and the receiver are relaxed and ready to begin, allow your leg to make contact. You will learn to sense when the time is right. Allow a few seconds of leg contact before proceeding to the next technique. Total time: 20 seconds.

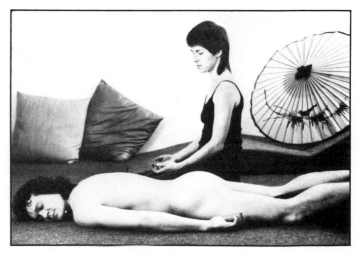

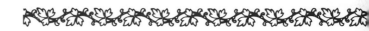

2) THE LAYING-ON OF HANDS

Purpose: The initial hand contact is of utmost importance. If compassion, sensitivity and confidence are expressed in the doer's hand, they will establish the proper tone and mood for the rest of the massage. Your hands must touch the receiver with authority and a gentle strength so that the receiver feels your hands are safe hands. Your initial contact should immediately secure the receiver's trust and submission in order for you to perform your part of the massage, which is GIVING. You cannot effectively give unless the receiver is willing to receive. The receiver must allow the doer to penetrate into the very essence of her/his being.

Positioning: Sit parallel to the receiver, Japanese style.

Procedure: Keep your leg in contact with the receiver's body as you proceed, very slowly and quietly, to *gently* lay one hand on the sacrum and then to lay the other directly over the spine between the scapulae (shoulder blades). Let your hands settle into the receiver's back the way butter melts into a pancake. When your hands are at full rest, your entire body should be relaxed. Maintain this contact for approximately 30 seconds. Be sure your wrists and hands are supple and relaxed, as tense hands will communicate tension to the receiver. Synchronize your breathing with the receiver's by audibly inhaling and ex-

haling at the receiver's rate at least five times. Then indicate to the receiver that you want to slow down the breathing rate by taking loud, deep, slow breaths. In a few seconds the receiver will sense your desire to relax and be one, and will usually sigh very deeply to indicate submission and readiness. Indeed, this deep sigh signifies the receiver is "in the now" of the massage, and you can proceed to the next technique, Spine Tracing.

Repetition: Repeat this technique only if you have been disturbed and must begin again.

Time: The entire technique will usually be accomplished in 60 seconds.

3) SPINE TRACING

Purpose: Spine Tracing relaxes the receiver and helps to eliminate superficial spinal tension. Spine Tracing also affords an excellent opportunity for the doer to make mental notes of hard, dry, puffy, flaky, scaly, hot or cold spots along the spine. These are the outward manifestations of inner disturbances. You will need to pay more attention to these spots when you begin Vertebrae Technique #6.

Positioning: Sit, Japanese style, as in Techniques #1 and #2.

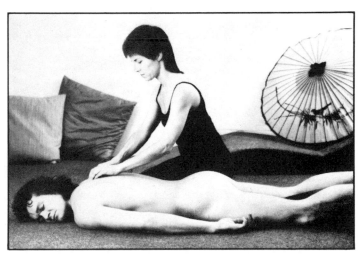

Procedure: Place three fingers on either side of the spine. Begin as close to the base of the skull as possible, and *very slowly,* with a medium pressure, pull your fingers all the way down either side of the spine. Continue over the sacrum and end at the tip of the coccyx. Remember to make mental notes of unusual muscle tension, skin textures or temperature changes of the skin along the spine.
Repetition: Repeat Spine Tracing two or three times.
Time: 40 seconds.

4) ROCKING THE BACK

Purpose: This technique serves further to loosen and relax the muscles of the back, as well as to prepare it for the heavy thumb pressure of Vertebrae Technique #5. It also feels very good.
Positioning: Sit, Japanese style, with your body perpendicular to the receiver's spine. The actual rocking motion will be performed in a slightly raised position.

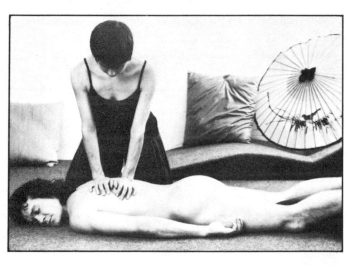

Procedure: Use the heels of your hands. Begin at the shoulders, one inch away from the spinal column. Holding your hands side by side, move them in unison back and forth in a rocking motion. As you proceed downward to the next area of the back, slightly overlap the area previously rocked in order to insure that no part of the back is neglected. Use your body weight to achieve the

rocking motion. *Do not use muscle power.* Rock all the way down to the sacrum. After you have completed one side, cross over the body and do the other side.
Repetition: Rock each area along the spine back and forth five times. Rock each side of the spine only once.
Time: 60 seconds.

5) DEEP BREATHING TECHNIQUE

Purpose: This technique helps the receiver release tension stored in the muscles of the back. It also relieves pressure on the nerves as they emerge from the spinal column.
Positioning: See Technique #6, Vertebrae Technique.
Procedure: Place your hands on either side of the spine near the neck. Ask the receiver to inhale. Then, as the receiver exhales, slowly allow your

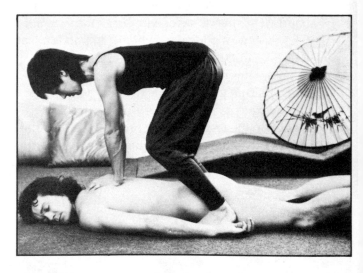

body weight to extend down your arms into your hands. Verbally encourage the receiver to exhale completely, for many people only partially exhale what they inhale. The pressure must be applied calmly so the receiver's back muscles don't tighten up in response to sudden pressure. Press when the receiver exhales as you continue down the spine to the coccyx.
Repetition: No repetition necessary.
Time: 30 seconds.

6) VERTEBRAE TECHNIQUE

Purpose: The Vertebrae Technique is executed in three phases.

PHASE	PURPOSE
1) Medium pressure, clockwise circular thumb massage.	Preparation for penetration by superficial relaxation of the back.
2) Firm penetrating pressure, executed with compassion, on either side of the spine. Use your thumbs.	Penetrating pressure releases tensions and triggers the body's natural healing mechanism.
3) Soothing, light, clockwise circular thumb massage.	"Making Nice." Alleviation of pain or discomfort caused by Phase 2:

Phase 3 of Vertebrae Technique is very important. It is essential to "make nice" because pain creates tension. By gently massaging the area affected, you encourage the receiver's body to release any pain or tension that has accumulated as a direct result of your firm thumb pressure in *Phase 2*. Remember, your aim is not to cause pain. You will, however, encounter areas that are tender or painful to the touch. Do not avoid these areas. Massage the sore spots. Be thorough, and be compassionate. Let your efforts be rewarded with the knowledge that the receiver's body will ultimately be experiencing less discomfort, improved energy and better blood circulation.

Positioning: There are three possible positions.

1) Straddle the receiver's body at the waist on your knees.

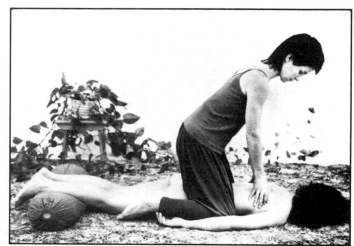

1)

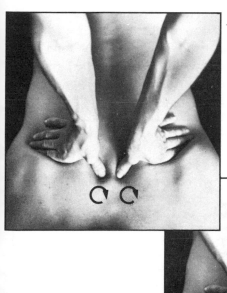

2)

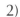

3)

59

2) Sit, Japanese style, at the receiver's side, parallel to the spine.

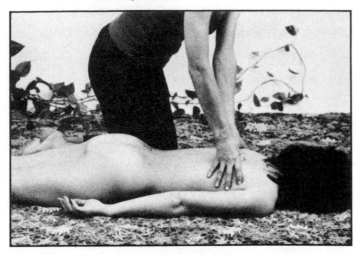

3) Stand, legs bent, straddling the receiver's body.

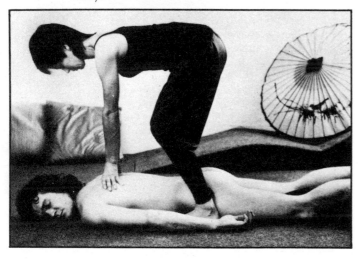

POSITION 1: is appropriate if the receiver is physically small enough for you to straddle. Do not sit or rest your body weight on the receiver.
POSITION 2: is used when the receiver is small enough for the doer to apply pressure evenly to both sides of the spinal column from one side of the body. As some people find Position 1 difficult to hold because their legs are spread apart, Position 2 is offered as an alternative. If you decide to use Position 2, be sure to apply equal pressure to both sides of the spinal column. Also, remember to keep your spine erect while you work. If you work in a slumped posture, you are very likely to strain your back muscles.
POSITION 3: is especially useful when the receiver is significantly larger than the doer. The extra height achieved in this raised position makes it easier for the doer to use body weight, rather than muscle power, to apply pressure. Position 3 also encourages equal distribution of body weight, because the doer is positioned directly over the receiver.
Procedure: Begin vertebrae massage and pressure on either side of and between the fifth and sixth thoracic vertebrae. See drawing.

There are two ways of locating the fifth and sixth thoracic vertebrae.

1) The lower tip of the scapula (shoulder blade) usually ends between the seventh and eighth intercostal space. Be sure the receiver's arms are stretched out at the side of the body, then count the spinous processes up from the base of the scapula to the fifth and sixth thoracic vertebrae.

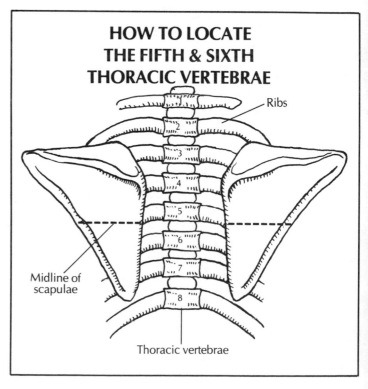

HOW TO LOCATE THE FIFTH & SIXTH THORACIC VERTEBRAE

Ribs

Midline of scapulae

Thoracic vertebrae

2) Eye-ball or approximate the location of the fifth and sixth thoracic by estimating the middle of the scapula. Midway between the top and bottom of the scapula is generally the location of the fifth and sixth thoracic vertebrae.

Once you have located the fifth and sixth thoracic vertebrae, begin implementing first *Phase 1,* then *Phase 2* and finally *Phase 3* on either side of and between each pair of the thoracic and lumbar vertebrae. There are twelve thoracic vertebrae, but for now you can ignore the first through the fifth, and there are five lumbar vertebrae. The lumbar vertebrae are located directly below the thoracic and terminate at the sacrum. Pressure must be applied perpendicularly to the plane of the body you are working. If the application of pressure is not perpendicular to the surface, the doer risks strained arms, sore thumbs or sudden back pain. Do not massage or apply pressure directly to the vertebral processes. This could prove painful or even damaging to the receiver. Reserve working on the upper thoracic vertebrae until you are seated at the receiver's head.

Repetition: PHASE 1: Use a medium pressure, clockwise circular thumb massage on either side of the spine between the vertebrae. Repeat rotations three to five times. If an area feels particularly tense, increase the number of rotations.

PHASE 2: Apply a firm penetrating pressure, executed with compassion, to either side of the spine between the transverse processes. The pressure is applied directly over the nerve as it emerges from the spinal column. Use your thumbs. If an area is particularly tense, release and repeat the pressure two or three times. Hold each application of pressure for 5 seconds.

PHASE 3: Use a light, soothing, clockwise circular thumb massaging motion. Repeat rotation three to five times, depending upon the intensity of the pain in that area when you were doing Phase 2.

Time: The entire mid and lower back will consume approximately five minutes of the massage. If the receiver is particularly tense, you will need to allot more time to complete this portion of the back.

7) SACRUM PRESSURE

Purpose: This technique relieves sacral tension and improves the flow of energy to the small intestines, bladder and sexual organs.

Positioning: There are three possible positions.

1) Sit parallel to the receiver's body.
2) Straddle the receiver's body on your knees.
3) Stand, legs bent, straddling the receiver.

Procedure: Locate the sacral foramina, the four holes on either side of the sacrum that transmit the sacral nerves and arteries. Once you have found these foramina, apply firm pressure to each of the depressions. Do both sides simultaneously.

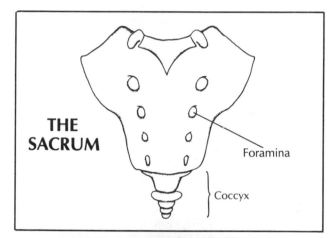

THE SACRUM — Foramina — Coccyx

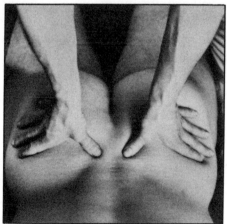

Repetition: No repetition is necessary, unless the receiver has a problem with either the small intestines, bladder or sexual organs.

Time: Hold the pressure over each of the foramina for 3-5 seconds. Total time: approximately 20 seconds.

8) BACK RELAXING & BROADENING STRETCH

Purpose: This technique suggests to the receiver's brain and back that you want the muscles of the back to broaden and relax. The stretch also feels very good.

Positioning: Same as #6, though Position 3 is most effective in this case, i.e. standing, legs bent, straddling the receiver's body.

Procedure: Begin by placing your thumbs on either side of the sacrum. Pull the thumbs out and away from the sacrum. Gently pulling the skin as

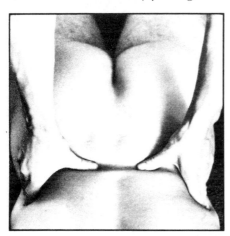

you move outward, slide the thumbs along the flesh and over the buttocks. Move up the sacrum one thumb space at a time, until you have covered the area entirely. Repeat the same technique, beginning on either side of and between the fourth and fifth lumbar vertebrae, and move up the back until you reach the neck.

Repetition: No repetition is necessary.

Time: Approximately 60 seconds.

9) WAIST & HIP LIFT

Purpose: This technique helps to trim the waistline. It also stimulates liver and gall bladder function.

Positioning: This technique is most efficiently done while straddling the receiver on your feet with your knees bent, but it can also be done while kneeling at the receiver's side.

Procedure: Slide your hands around and under

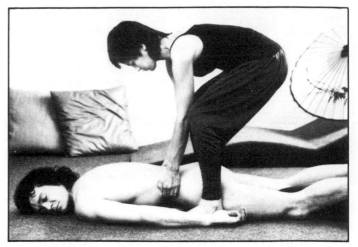

the receiver's waist. Holding the waist firmly, pull up with your hands. If the receiver is small-boned and not overweight, you may actually be able to lift the body slightly off the mat. It is not necessary to achieve this lift. It is only necessary to lift the flesh of the waist. If you can manage it easily, however, don't hesitate to lift the body up off the mat. Then, grasping the hip bones, lift the hips and buttocks off the mat.

Repetition: Lift the waist and hips twice.

Time: 30 seconds.

10) KNEADING OF THE BUTTOCKS

Purpose: Pressure and massage of the buttocks area is beneficial to the sciatic nerve, which is the largest nerve in the body. You are also massaging the gluteus maximus and gluteus medius muscles. Applied Kinesiology has proven that specific muscles correspond to particular organs. The gluteals correspond to the sexual and reproductive organs. The condition of these muscles can influence the general health and functioning of their related organs. For example, people who have weak or flabby gluteus muscles will often have ovary, uterus, womb or prostate problems. As these muscles often are flabby, they need massage to tone the loose flesh and improve the energy flow to the sexual and reproductive organs.

Positioning: Straddle the receiver's legs on your knees. Keep your spine in the correct alignment as your work.

Procedure : Two basic techniques accomplish the desired results.

1) With the heels of your hands begin a light to medium circular massaging motion. The buttocks is very often tender or painful, so work with great compassion. Massage the entire buttocks area twice to prepare adequately for your subsequent firm heel pressure.

2) Apply a slow, firm pressure with the heel of your hand to the entire buttocks area. Apply the pressure gradually so that you will know if the receiver is beginning to feel pain. Do not apply pressure if it causes too much pain. A little "good" pain helps to release the tension and/or blockage, but you don't need to torture the receiver. When your pressure begins to cause some discomfort, discontinue further penetration and hold pressure for 5 seconds. The area will become less painful as the seconds pass, and the tension or energy blockage will be relieved to some extent. Chronic sciatic conditions require more applications of pressure than acute conditions.

Repetition: Technique 1: Massage the entire buttocks area several times.
Technique 2: Slowly apply firm heel-of-the-hand pressure to five different locations on the buttocks. Hold pressure 5 seconds.
Time: Allow approximately 30 seconds for massaging and 25 seconds for the heel-of-the-hand technique.

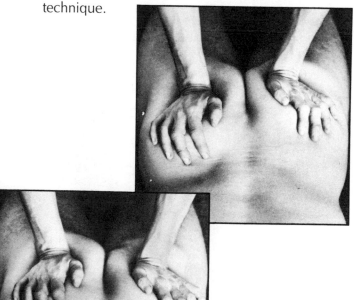

BACKS OF THE LEGS

When massaging the backs of the legs, you will be applying pressure to the Bladder Meridian. Stimulation of this meridian will help the body to correct bladder conditons. Frequent urination, frequent desire with scanty emission and pain during urination are some of the conditions known to respond to Bladder Meridian pressure. If you have a bladder or urinary tract infection, pressure applied to this meridian will encourage the body's natural healing mechanism to work more quickly. The Bladder Meridian also affects the functioning of the kidney hormone system, as well as the autonomic nervous system of the urinary and reproductive organs.

11) THIGH BLADDER MERIDIAN PRESSURE

Purpose: This technique relaxes the back of the legs and affects the Bladder Meridian.
Positioning: Kneel between the receiver's legs.
Procedure: Use the heels of your hands. Begin to apply pressure below the gluteus maximus

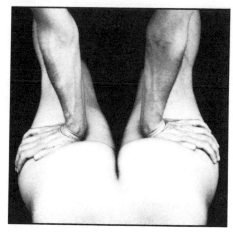

muscle, i.e. just below the buttocks. Do both legs at the same time, but alternate the firm pressure between the left heel and right heel of your hands as you move down the back of the leg to the crease of the knee. Hold each application of pressure 3-5 seconds.
Repetition: No repetition necessary.
Time: 20 seconds.

12) CREASE OF THE KNEE ACUPUNCTURE PRESSURE POINTS

Purpose: This technique effects a positive change in the Bladder Meridian and its related functions. It also releases tension stored in the knee.
Positioning: Kneel between the receiver's legs.
Procedure: Use your thumbs. Apply a firm, gentle and steady pressure to the center of the back of the crease of the knees. Keep your back aligned.

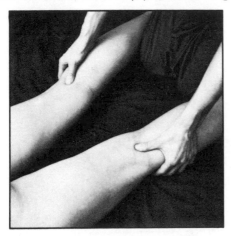

Repetition: Repeat the application of pressure three times and hold each for 3 seconds.
Time: Approximately 10 seconds.

13) LOWER BACK OF THE LEG BLADDER MERIDIAN PRESSURE

Purpose: Pressure here affects the Bladder Meridian and helps to relax the calf muscle. As the gastrocnemius, or calf muscle, correlates to the adrenal glands in Applied Kinesiology, you are also strengthening the functioning of the receiver's adrenal glands.
Positioning: Kneel between the receiver's legs.
Procedure: Use the heels of your hands to apply a slow, firm pressure down the center back of the calf muscle. The belly of the muscle, its widest part, cannot tolerate as much pressure as the rest of the leg. Be careful with your pressure here. Reduce it by half at the belly of the gastrocnemius.
Repetition: No repetition necessary.
Time: 20 seconds.

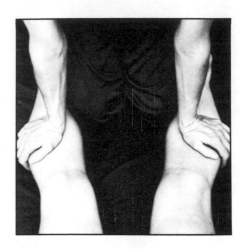

14) ACHILLES TENDON SQUEEZE

Purpose: Squeezing the Achilles tendon affects the prostate, uterus and rectum, as well as chronic sciatic nerve conditions. It also helps to strengthen and relax the calf muscle. The adrenal glands, which are related to the calf muscle, are also affected.
Positioning: Sit, Japanese style, at the receiver's feet.
Procedure: Squeeze the entire length of the Achilles tendon by using the index finger and the thumb. As you continue up the calf, to just above the knee joint, squeeze the large muscles of the lower leg.
Repetition: Squeeze the entire length of the Achilles tendon and the calf to just above the knee joint twice.
Time: Hold each squeeze for 3 seconds. The entire technique done twice, will take 30 seconds.

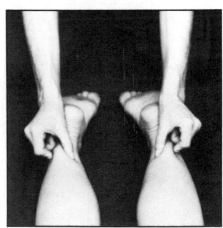

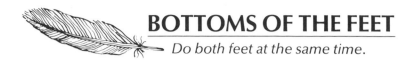

BOTTOMS OF THE FEET
Do both feet at the same time.

15) BOTTOM OF THE FOOT ACKNOWLEDGMENT

Purpose: This technique loosens the feet and prepares them for specific pressure point therapy.
Positioning: Sit, Japanese style, at receiver's feet.
Procedure: Use your thumbs to firmly massage the entire bottoms of the receiver's feet. Let your thumbs move freely. Keep them flexible and

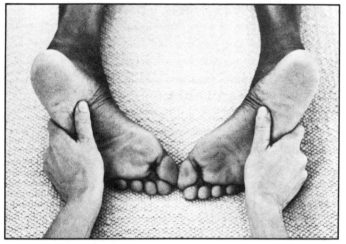

in constant motion. Do not get specific with this technique. It is a general massage technique designed primarily to relax the feet before specific pressure point therapy.
Repetition: Two or three times.
Time: 30 seconds.

16) HEEL TWIST

Purpose: This technique helps to stimulate the flow of fresh blood into the feet and to release tension from the feet and ankles.

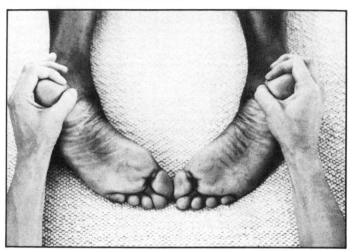

Positioning: Sit at the receiver's feet.
Procedure: Grasp both heels, hold them firmly, and simultaneously twist them first inward and then outward.
Repetition: Repeat three times in each direction.
Time: 10 seconds.

It is important to be familiar with the skeletal structure of the feet when applying heavy pressure.

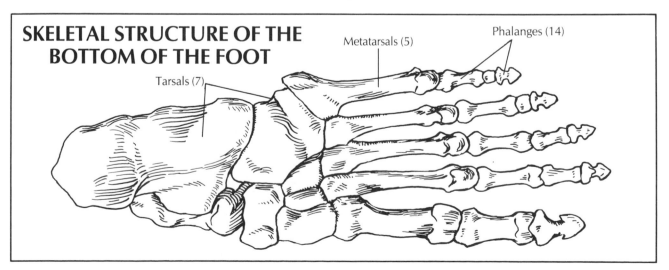

SKELETAL STRUCTURE OF THE BOTTOM OF THE FOOT

Tarsals (7)

Metatarsals (5)

Phalanges (14)

17) SQUEEZE & TWIST EDGE OF FOOT

Purpose: This regenerates the nervous system.
Positioning: Sit, at the receiver's feet.
Procedure: Begin this technique near the heel of the outside edge of the foot, and then continue

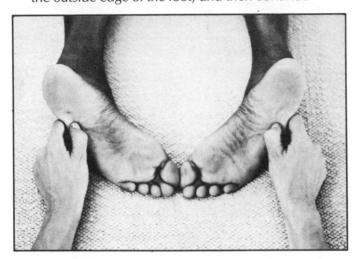

down the edge of the foot to the toes. Take some flesh between your thumb and index finger. Squeeze and gently twist the skin.
Repetition: None.
Time: 10 seconds.

18) OUTER EDGE OF THE FOOT PRESSURE

Purpose: This technique regenerates the nervous system. It is also helpful with shoulder, arm, elbow, hip and knee conditions. Hemorrhoids, too, respond to pressure applied to the back of the heel. Many people feel tingles up and down the spine during this technique. This feeling is the movement of nerve energy along the spinal column.

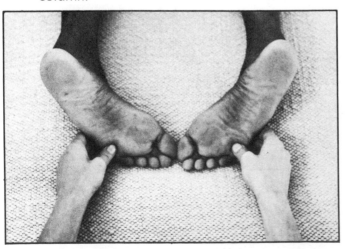

Positioning: Sit, at the receiver's feet.
Procedure: Apply a firm penetrating thumb pressure to both feet at the same time. Begin under the small toe and work your way up and around to the heel.
Repetition: Unnecessary.
Time: Hold each pressure point for 3-5 seconds. The entire technique will take 35 seconds.

19) BOTTOMS OF THE FEET PRESSURE POINTS

Purpose: Pressure applied to the related organ points on the soles of the feet stimulates the nerve endings, which, in turn, stimulate the entire nerve and its associated organs and muscles. This stimulation encourages the body's natural healing mechanism to take control and begins to right most conditions of ill health. The toxins that accumulate in the feet are released, and the general health and condition of the nerves are improved. So is the overall health of the receiver.
Positioning: Sit, at the receiver's feet.
Procedure: Apply firm pressure with your thumbs or knuckles to each of the diagnostic points. Hold pressure for 3-5 seconds. When applying pressure, direct your thoughts to the organ related to the reflex point. Try to visualize the organ. Concentration will accomplish greater results than will an absent-minded pressure.
Repetition: If any of the reflex points feels painful or tender, repeat the pressure on that point. The repetition must be gentler than the first application. The purpose is to soothe the area and give the tender reflex point the one more application of pressure needed to complete the triggering of the body's natural healing mechanism.
Time: 60 seconds.

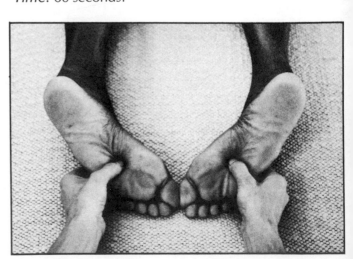

F O O T   R E F L E X O L O G Y

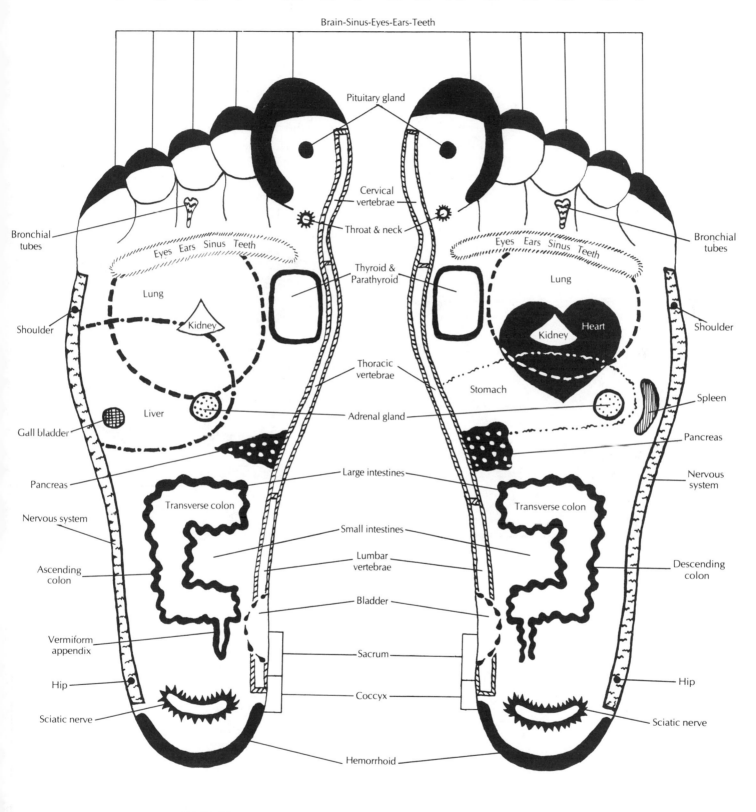

Brain-Sinus-Eyes-Ears-Teeth

Pituitary gland

Cervical vertebrae

Throat & neck

Bronchial tubes

Eyes Ears Sinus Teeth

Thyroid & Parathyroid

Lung

Shoulder

Kidney

Thoracic vertebrae

Liver

Adrenal gland

Gall bladder

Pancreas

Large intestines

Nervous system

Transverse colon

Ascending colon

Small intestines

Lumbar vertebrae

Vermiform appendix

Bladder

Hip

Sacrum

Sciatic nerve

Coccyx

Hemorrhoid

Eyes Ears Sinus Teeth

Lung

Heart

Kidney

Stomach

Spleen

Pancreas

Nervous system

Transverse colon

Descending colon

Bladder

Hip

Sciatic nerve

Bronchial tubes

Shoulder

RIGHT

LEFT

67

20) TOE PAD PRESSURE, MASSAGE & SQUEEZE

Purpose: Massaging and squeezing the toes improves sinus conditions and relieves brain fatigue. Slow learners or mentally overworked individuals will benefit from this technique.

Positioning: Sit, at the receiver's feet.

Procedure: Use your thumbs to apply a firm pressure to the pads of the toes. Begin with the little toe on each foot, then work your way toward the big toe. Squeeze the sides, top and bottom of each toe.

Repetition: Repeat these techniques if the receiver is frequently troubled with sinus conditions or brain fatigue.

Time: 45 seconds.

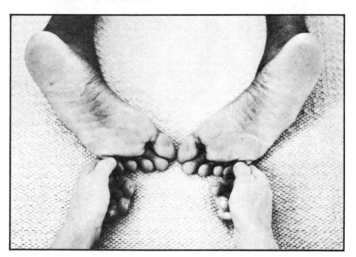

21) HEEL PRESSURE FOR SCIATIC NERVE

Purpose: This technique relieves sciatic nerve pain.

Positioning: Sit at the receiver's feet.

Procedure: Apply heavy thumb or knuckle pressure to the middle of the heel area.

Repetition: Repeat as often as necessary to relieve acute pain. If there is no pain but you wish to help cure a chronic sciatic condition, apply pressure four times to each heel.

Time: Hold each pressure point 3-5 seconds, for a total of approximately 15 seconds.

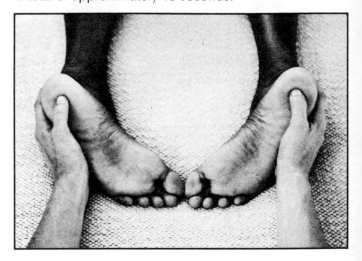

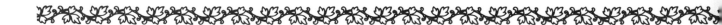

SHOULDERS AND UPPER BACK

22) SHOULDER SHRUG

Purpose: Use in alternation with Technique #23 to encourage the relaxation of the shoulder and upper arm muscles.

Positioning: Sit at receiver's head.

Procedure: Massage the deltoid muscle, then grasp the top of the arms and pull the shoulders

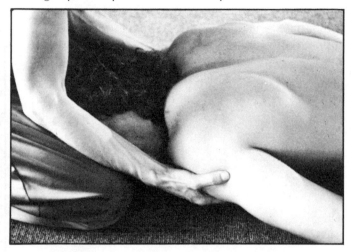

up toward the head. Use Shoulder Slide Technique #23 to return the shoulders to their normal position.

Repetition: Repeat the Shoulder Shrug two times, but alternate each shrug with Technique #23.

Time: See Technique #23.

23) SHOULDER SLIDE

Purpose: Most people hold their shoulders somewhere in the vicinity of their ears. This may be a slight exaggeration, but the fact is that many people do have a great deal of tension stored in their shoulders. Eventually, chronic neck and shoulder tension will permanently alter one's posture. The Shoulder Slide returns the shoulders to their correct position. This technique also enables the receiver to become aware of how high the shoulders are normally held.

Positioning: Sit at the receiver's head. Crouch so that the pressure does not strain your shoulders, but keep your spine properly aligned.

Procedure: Cradle the receiver's shoulders in the palms of your hands. Slowly slide the shoulders

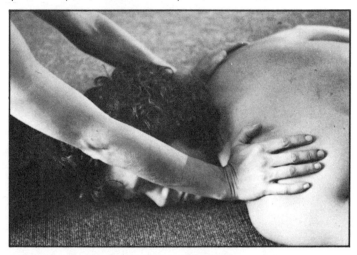

down toward the feet. Hold the shoulders in the full stretch position for 5 seconds.

Repetition: Repeat two times in alternation with Technique #22.

Time: 15 seconds.

24) SHOULDER ROTATIONS

Purpose: Shoulder Rotations relax the upper trapezius muscle and the muscles of the shoulder. They thereby release tension from the neck and the shoulders.

Positioning: There are two possible positions to assume.

1) Sit, Japanese style, at the receiver's head.
2) Kneel parallel to the receiver's body in the vicinity of the waist.

Procedure: If you assume *Position 1*, grasp both shoulders and rotate them toward you. Lift the receiver's shoulders off the mat during the motion. If the receiver is of normal weight and delicate-boned, you will be able to rotate both shoulders simultaneously.

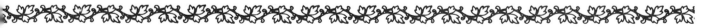

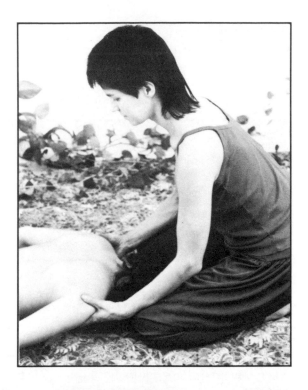

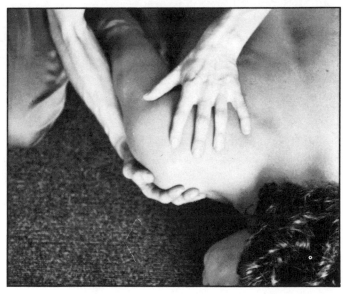

If you assume *Position 2,* slide one arm under the receiver's arm and shoulder. Use your other hand to cup the same shoulder. Now, use your arms and hands to rotate the shoulder. Rotate clockwise and counter-clockwise three times in each direction. Repeat procedure on receiver's other shoulder.
Repetition: If the receiver has chronic shoulder tension or pain, increase the number of rotations.
Time: Allow 5 seconds.

25) UPPER THORACIC VERTEBRAE TECHNIQUE

Purpose: This technique relaxes the muscles of the upper back and shoulders. The lungs, thyroid, eyes, ears, heart and stomach benefit greatly from the applications of this procedure. Also, pressure is relieved on the nerves as they emerge from the spinal column.
Positioning: Sit, Japanese style, at the receiver's head.
Procedure: Begin on either side of and between the fourth and fifth thoracic vetebrae. Execute in the same three phases as Technique #6, Vertebrae Technique.

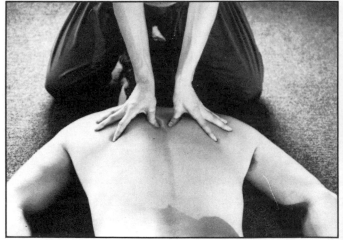

Repetition:
Phase 1: Massage between and on either side of the vertebrae three to five times by applying medium pressure with your thumbs.
Phase 2: Apply thumb pressure for 3-5 seconds to the same areas. If an area is particularly painful, repeat pressure.
Phase 3: Massage the same areas three to five times with your thumbs applying light pressure. "Make Nice."
See the photographs for Technique #6 on page 59
Time: 60 seconds.

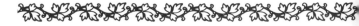

26) UPPER TRAPEZIUS SHOULDER PRESS

Purpose: The upper trapezius, the most prominent muscle of the shoulder, is often weak or tense. This technique is designed to release tension from this muscle.

Positioning: Sit, Japanese style, at the receiver's head. Lower your torso in order to facilitate the correct application of the pressure.

Procedure: Begin at the outer edge of the shoulders, between the clavicle and the spine of the scapula. Use thumb pressure along the fullest part

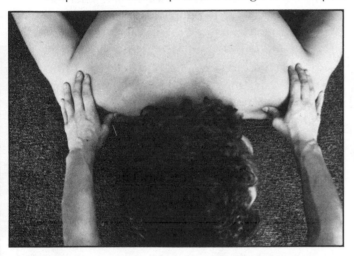

of the muscle. Work your way from the edge of the shoulders toward the vertebrae of the neck. Return to the outer edge of the shoulders. Repeat the thumb pressure along the same area. The pressure must be firm and sensitive. Most people will experience pain with these points. Do not jab your thumbs into the muscle tissue. Penetrate slowly and firmly.

Repetition: If the receiver experiences chronic shoulder tension, repeat this technique after Technique #27.

Time: Hold each thumb application of pressure for 3-5 seconds. The entire technique will take 25 seconds.

27) UPPER TRAPEZIUS SHOULDER SQUEEZE & MASSAGE

Purpose: The Shoulder Squeeze improves the flow of blood to the muscles being massaged and releases pockets of tension. It feels very good.

Positioning: Sit, Japanese style, at the receiver's head.

Procedure: Using your fingers and thumbs, massage with great compassion because a great deal of tension is stored in the shoulders. If a puffy, lumpy area comes to your attention, you have

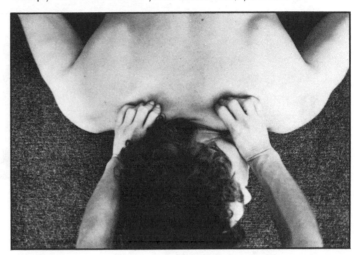

found an energy blockage or tension pocket. Concentrate on these areas, and alternate a gentle massaging motion with a delicate squeezing one. Energy blockages or tension pockets can also be dispersed by applying a gentle, but firm thumb pressure directly to the site of the blockage.

Repetition: Thumb pressure applied directly to the site of a blockage must be held for 5-7 seconds. Repeat massaging and squeezing many times.

Time: The entire technique, including massaging, thumb pressure and squeezing, will require 30 seconds.

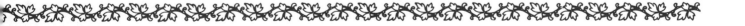

28) SHOULDER KNEADING

Purpose: Kneading releases tension and helps to free blockages in the shoulders.
Positioning: Sit, Japanese style, at receiver's head.
Procedure: Use the heels of both of your hands. Knead the part of the shoulders that is farthest

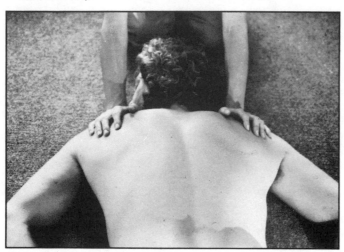

from the neck by alternating your pressure from the right to left heel. Knead *slowly* so that the rhythm established feels like a rocking, soothing motion.
Repetition: Knead each shoulder a total of five times.
Time: 10 seconds.

29) SPINAL SWEEP

Purpose: This technique provides a nice farewell to the spine before moving on to the feet. The Spinal Sweep is very relaxing.

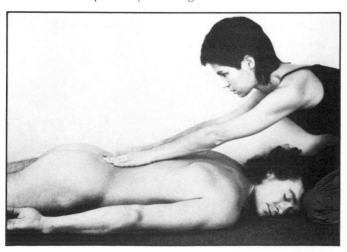

Positioning: Sit, Japanese style, at the receiver's head.
Procedure: Lay both hands flat on the sacrum. Using a medium pressure, pull your hands up along either side of the spine. As your hands reach the neck, use a lighter motion to continue the stroke up and over the neck and head.
Repetition: Repeat three times.
Time: 20 seconds.

30) FEATHERING THE SPINE

Purpose: The light gliding motion of feathering often produces goose pimples in the receiver. Feathering tells the brain to relax the area that is being feathered. Feathering is also a very quiet and gentle way to leave one part of the body for another so that the massage can continue without abrupt loss of contact.
Positioning: Sit, Japanese style, at receiver's head.
Procedure: Feather directly over the spine. Begin feathering with the right hand, then alternate with the left. Feather three inches along the coccyx with the right hand. Begin the next stroke with the left hand, but overlap by approximately one inch the area you have just feathered with the right. As you proceed, always overlap the previous area so that no part of the spine is neglected. Be sure to continue the feathering over the neck and head. Visualize that you are pulling energy up the Governing Meridian, which affects the entire spine and nervous system.
Repetition: Repeat the entire feathering of the spine two times. Complete the technique with your hands lightly resting on the receiver's head.
Time: 20 seconds.

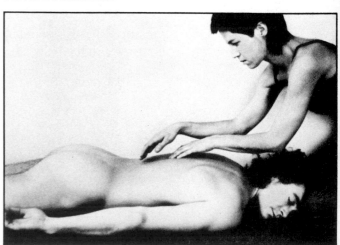

LYING SUPINE

When Technique #30 has been completed, allow 15-20 seconds for the receiver to lie comfortably relaxed. Remain seated, Japanese style, continue to hold the receiver's head loosely with both hands. Then, over a period of 30 seconds, slowly, gradually and imperceptibly draw your hands away from the head. The withdrawal must be slow so that you do not startle the receiver. This gradual departure from the body leaves the receiver feeling calm, safe and often asleep. Use a light touch and a soft voice to bring the receiver back from a sleep state. Suggest that the receiver turn over when ready and able. Even if the receiver is not asleep, use this method to leave the body and reestablish verbal communication.

A few adjustments must be made to assure the receiver's comfort while lying supine.

A) Place one folded bed pillow under each leg. The pillow raises the legs slightly and thus takes pressure off the lower back. People who suffer from chronic low back pain will appreciate the relief. Those who do not will receive a more relaxed massage.

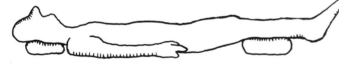

B) Squat at the receiver's head. Place both hands and arms under the shoulders and partially under the back. Take hold of the back and stretch it toward you. Stretching the spine eliminates the exaggerated arch of the lower back, which is the result of weak abdominals and tense lower back muscles. Stretching and flattening the back allows it to assume a more correct alignment. Receiving

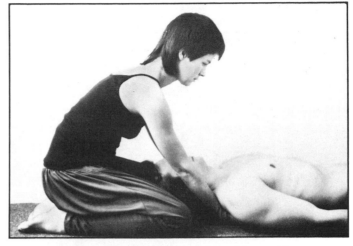

a massage in a stretched, relaxed position with the spine properly aligned enables the body to release more tension.

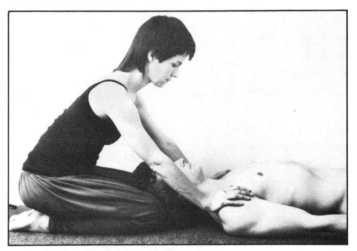

C) Cup the shoulders and push them down toward the receiver's toes.

D) Grasp the underside of the receiver's head and neck, then stretch and pull the head and neck toward you. Repeat this stretching and pulling three times.

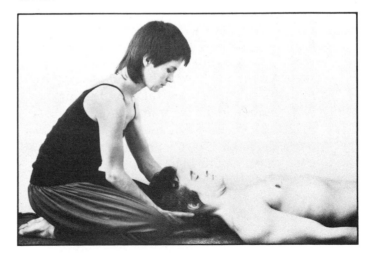

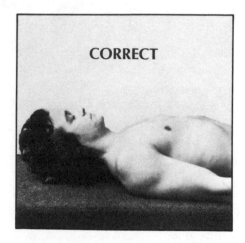

CORRECT

E) Next, raise the head slightly and insert a thin pillow under the occipital protuberance, which is the big bump at the back of the head. If you do not have a tiny pillow, use a towel that has been folded tightly. The aim is to raise the head about 1¹/₂-2 inches off the mat. The following photograph shows that when the head lies on the mat, it tends to tilt up and back. This tilt puts pressure on

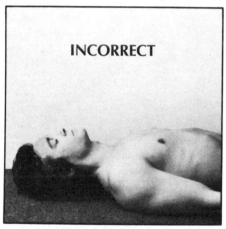

INCORRECT

the first few cervical vertebrae and increases tension in the shoulders and neck. Once the head is on the pillow, insert your fingers under the base of the skull and again stretch the neck toward you. Rest the receiver's head, with the neck in the stretched position, on the pillow. Be sure the chin is not sticking up in the air. In this position much of the tension in the neck and shoulders will automatically be released as you massage the rest of the body. Indeed, by the time you begin massaging the neck, much of the blockage and pain has already been relieved.

F) Cover the receiver if the possibility of a chill exists. Use a sheet in warm weather and an electric blanket when the air is cool or cold.

G) If the receiver feels any tension or pain in the neck or shoulders as a result of lying in the prone position for the back work, massage the neck and shoulders for one or two minutes by using Techniques #69 and #71. These techniques will release any discomfort and allow you to proceed to THE FEET PART II.
Time: 4 minutes.

TOP OF THE FEET

31) GENERAL FOOT ACKNOWLEDGMENT (BOTH FEET)

Purpose: This technique loosens and relaxes the feet before the application of specific pressure point techniques. A brief, gentle massage before beginning to apply heavy pressure enables the feet to enjoy the firmer pressure.
Positioning: Sit, at the receiver's feet.
Procedure: Acknowledge the entire foot by massaging it with gentle pressure and by lightly stroking and bending the foot.
Repetition: Unnecessary
Time: 30 seconds.

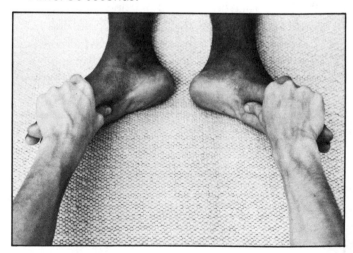

32) PULL AND MASSAGE TOES (BOTH FEET)

Purpose: Massaging and pulling the toes helps to loosen each toe. This technique also returns stagnant blood to the heart and thus allows fresh blood to flow to the toes. When you consider the shoes we wear, especially those worn by women, it is easy to understand why massaging and pulling the toes feels so good and relieves so much pain. Manipulation of the toes also indirectly moves the metatarsal bones and helps to loosen the bones and muscles of the foot itself. Furthermore, toe manipulation helps to improve sinus conditions and brain fatigue as well as other brain-related conditions.

Positioning: Remain seated, Japanese style, at the feet.

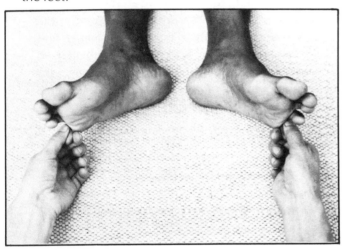

Procedure: Begin massaging the small toes. Methodically, toe by toe, work your way to the big toes. Manipulate the same toes on each foot at the same time. Squeeze and massage each toe from the tip of its nail to the base where it joins the foot. Massaging from the base of the toe to the tip of the nail does not return as much stagnant blood to the heart for recirculation. After you have massaged one pair of toes, give the same toes a firm, but gentle pull and twist to stretch and further relax them.

Repetition: Unnecessary.

Time: Allow 10 seconds for each pair of toes. The total time will be approximately 50 seconds.

33) ANKLE ROTATIONS (ONE FOOT)

Purpose: These rotations relax the joint and increase the flexibility of the ankle. In addition to improving blood and lymph circulation, this technique frees stagnant meridian energy trapped in the ankles.

Positioning: Sit, Japanese style, at the receiver's side. Position yourself perpendicular to the calf muscles.

Procedure: Grasp the ball of the foot. Rest the receiver's lower leg over your knees. Be sure the ankle and foot do not make contact with your legs. With the palm of one hand, hold the bottom of the receiver's foot. With your other hand, support the leg just above the ankle. Make three large, slow rotations, first to the right and then to the left.

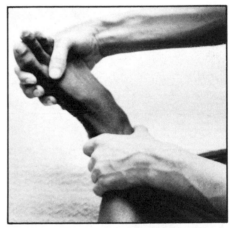

Repetition: Complete all three rotations in one direction before rotating in the other direction.

Time: 10 seconds per foot.

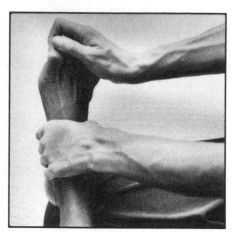

34) FIVE-TOE ROTATION (ONE FOOT)

Purpose: This technique further loosens cramped toes and metatarsal bones.

Positioning: Same as technique #33.

Procedure: Grasp the foot with one hand and hold the toes with the other hand. Slowly rotate all five toes at once.

Repetition: Rotate three times to the right and then to the left.

Time: 5 seconds per foot.

35) INDIVIDUAL TOE ROTATIONS AND PULLS (ONE FOOT)

Purpose: This technique continues to loosen cramped and tense toes. It also improves sinus conditions and brain fatigue.

Positioning: Same as technique #33.

Procedure: Rotate each toe. Rotate it in both directions, and then pull the toe firmly while twisting it slightly. You may hear a popping sound coming from the toes. This is a good sound, for it indicates that the toe joint has been released. Most people enjoy toe rotations and pulls, although some find it very unpleasant and even

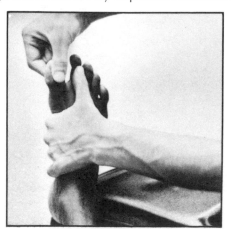

painful. If you sense discomfort on the part of the receiver, *gently* rotate and *lightly* stretch the toes. Do not force them to tolerate a more firmly executed pull and twist. Remember that pain is not the object and that excellent results can be achieved without causing excess discomfort.

Repetition: Rotate each toe twice in both directions, then twist as you pull. If you do not get the desired popping sound, try to pull the toe once more. If, however, it does not come easily the second time, move on to the next toe.

Time: Allow approximately 10 seconds per toe and a total of 50 seconds per foot.

36) ARCH PRESSURE FOR THE SPINE (ONE FOOT)

Purpose: Pressure along the arch of the foot helps to relieve back pain. Tension and spasms both respond quite quickly to these reflex points. If the receiver experiences occasional back pain, but is not feeling pain at the time of the massage, this technique will help discourage the return of the pain. Also it will ultimately help to correct the condition. Acute back pain, the sort that occurs suddenly because of a fall or because of lifting a heavy object, responds very well to these pressure points. Pressure along the arch of the foot also helps to rejuvenate the entire nervous system.

Positioning: Sit, Japanese style, at the receiver's head.

Procedure: Apply firm pressure from the outside base of the big toe nail, then along the arch of the foot to the back of the heel. Use the tip of your

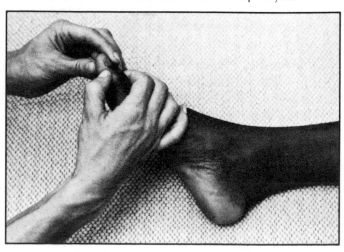

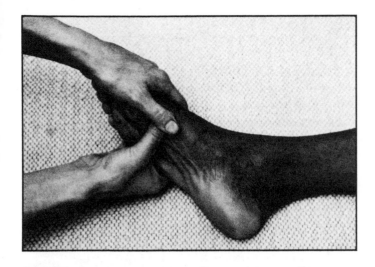

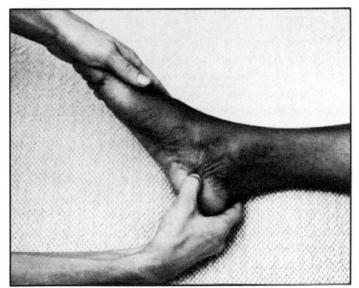

37) KIDNEY & SEXUAL/
REPRODUCTIVE ORGANS
MASSAGE (ONE FOOT)

Purpose: Points corresponding to the kidneys and sexual organs are located in approximately the same place. Pressure applied to the appropriate area will assist the kidneys in their eliminative processes and will tone up the sexual organs of both males and females. Reproductive, menstrual, prostate and other sexual organ malfunctioning can be corrected by regular applications of pressure to these reflex points.

Positioning: Sit, Japanese style, at the receiver's feet.

Procedure: Holding one of the receiver's feet in your hand, apply several applications of firm pressure to the hollow area just below the inside of the anklebone.

Repetition: Repeat only if the receiver has any condition that these points will help.

Time: Approximately 10 seconds per foot.

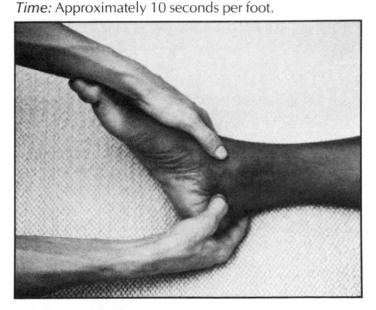

thumb to apply firm pressure from the base of the nail until you pass the sesamoid bone, which is the large bony protrusion on the bottom of the foot under the big toe. Next, using the ball of one thumb and assisting with your other thumb, apply firm, lingering pressure from the sesamoid bone to the heel. Use the tip-of-the-thumb technique for the heel. Don't skip any area of the arch. Apply pressure to every inch of the entire area discussed.

Repetition: If the receiver has back pain when you begin the massage, several applications will be necessary to relieve it. Otherwise, once down the toe, arch and heel is sufficient.

Time: Hold each pressure application for 3-5 seconds. Total time amounts to 50 seconds per foot.

38) ANKLEBONE MASSAGE (ONE FOOT)

Purpose: Massaging directly around the anklebone will benefit the male and female reproductive organs. It also feels really nice.

Positioning: Sit, Japanese style, at the receiver's feet.

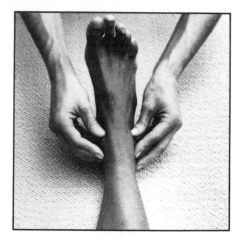

Procedure: Cup the fingers and thumb of each hand around the anklebones of one foot. Massage the area by moving all the fingers and your thumbs in unison. Stay close to the anklebone.

Repetition: Repeat only if the receiver's condition warrants continued use of these points.

Time: 5 seconds per foot.

39) ANKLE LYMPHATIC MASSAGE (BOTH FEET)

Purpose: This procedure flushes the lymphatic system at the ankle and moves along the stagnant toxins. Lymph tends to stagnate in the feet because most of us lead sedentary lives and have poor circulation

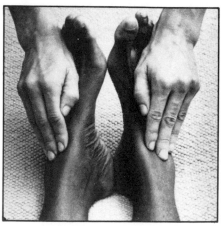

Positioning: Sit, Japanese style, at the receiver's feet.

Procedure: Use four fingers in a back-and-forth motion. Put most of your force in the forward motion so that the toxins will flush away from the feet. Gently bring your fingers back in preparation for the next motion forward. Do both feet at the same time.

Repetition: Use five firm motions backed up with five light gliding motions.

Time: 5 seconds.

40) FOUR FINGER METATARSAL SLIDE (BOTH FEET)

Purpose: Sliding your fingers along the grooves of the metatarsal bones is a very pleasurable sensation. This technique sends energy to the chest, lung and breast area. Any condition relating to this area of the body will heal itself more quickly with repeated use of these points.

Positioning: Sit, Japanese style, at the receiver's feet.

Procedure: Position the four fingers of both hands in the grooves of the metatarsal bones at the base of the toes on the top of both feet. Firmly force your fingers into these grooves while slowly and firmly sliding them toward and over the ankle. The technique is more pleasurable if the motion continues up and over the ankle. As the metatarsal bones do not extend to the ankle, you will loosen the grooves, but the pleasurable skin sensations derived from the pressure of the fingers sliding up and over the ankle warrants its continuation.

Repetition: Repeat three times on both feet at the same time.

Time: A total of 10 seconds is required.

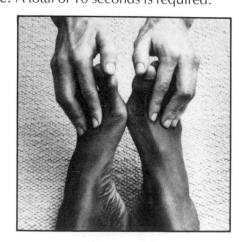

41) TOP OF THE FOOT TWIST (ONE FOOT)

Purpose: This twist relaxes the foot.
Positioning: Sit between the receiver's feet.
Procedure: Grasping the foot with both hands, twist your hands in opposite directions up and down the foot.

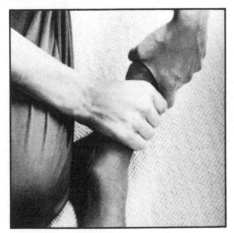

Repetition: Twist the entire foot twice.
Time: 7 seconds per foot.

At this point you have completed a thorough massage of one foot. Repeat Techniques #33 through #38, and #41, on the other foot. Then proceed to Technique #42.

FOOT REFLEXOLOGY SIDE VIEWS

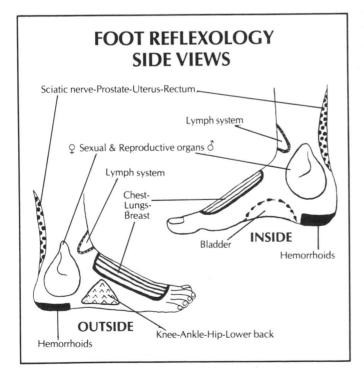

Sciatic nerve-Prostate-Uterus-Rectum

Lymph system

♀ Sexual & Reproductive organs ♂

Lymph system

Chest-Lungs-Breast

INSIDE

Bladder

Hemorrhoids

OUTSIDE

Hemorrhoids

Knee-Ankle-Hip-Lower back

FRONT OF THE LEGS

42) LIVER AID

Purpose: Applying pressure to the liver points along the shinbone will assist the liver in the performance of its 500 known functions. An extremely overworked organ, the liver can use all the help it can get. People who drink a lot of alcohol will find these points particularly useful.
Positioning: Sit, Japanese style, slightly between the receiver's legs.
Procedure: Begin at the ankle. Apply firm 3-second thumb pressure in the designated places as you move up the shinbone.

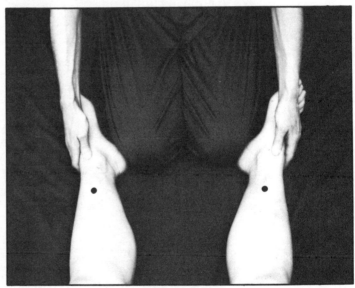

Repetition: No repetition is necessary unless a known liver condition or weakness exists. In such a case, repeat pressure to all the points three times and hold each point for ten seconds.
Time: 10 seconds, if no known condition exists.

43) KNEE LYMPHATIC MASSAGE

Purpose: This technique clears the lymph nodes that cluster around the knee and helps to strengthen the tendons of the muscles that insert around the knee. Knee pain also responds to this technique.

Positioning: Sit, Japanese style, between the receiver's open legs.

Procedure: Using four fingers and a circular massaging motion, massage around both knees at the same time. If knee problems exist, use firm thumb pressure on the same area after the four-finger massage. Do not directly massage the patella, or knee cap, as this does not feel good to the receiver. When applying firm thumb pressure, penetrate slowly so that you can clearly determine the bony structure under the skin. If pressure is ap-

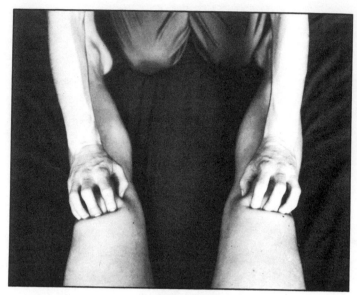

plied too quickly, you will not be fully aware of the underlying bone structure and may very well slip and hurt the receiver.

Repetition: Massage each area with four fingers five times. When applying thumb pressure, hold each pressure application for 3-5 seconds.

Time: 30 seconds.

44) THIGH LYMPHATIC FLUSH

Purpose: The Thigh Lymphatic Flush is useful for several conditions. Primarily it improves the functioning of the small and large intestines as well as that of the sexual and reproductive organs. Massaging the inside of the thigh also affects the tone and functioning of the abdominal muscles, the hamstrings and the quadratus lumborum. Low back pain, headaches and hemorrhoids also respond to thigh massage and manipulation. Massaging the outside of the thigh helps to alleviate breast and chest pain before, during and after menstruation. It is also very stimulating and beneficial to the colon. Constipation, diarrhea and other colon conditions respond favorably to the massaging of these points on a regular basis.

Positioning: Kneel below the receiver's knee with your knees on either side of the receiver's leg. Do not sit on the leg, for it may be uncomfortable for the receiver to bear the pressure of your body weight.

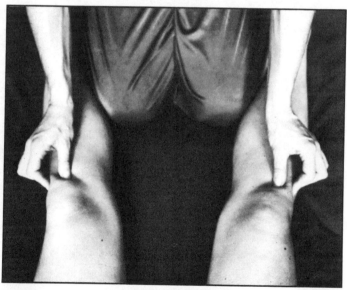

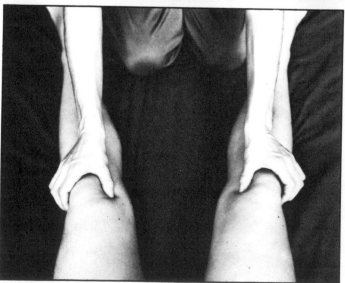

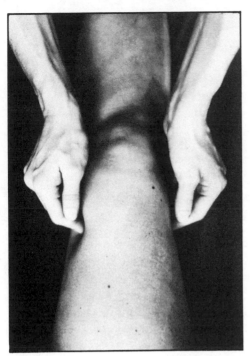

Procedure: Place four fingers of each hand on either side of one thigh beside the knee. Massage one leg at a time. Use a progressive, circular massaging motion as you work your way up the thigh. Use medium to firm pressure. Proceed with great compassion, for this area is very often tender.

Repetition: Repeat two times, more often if a problem relating to these lymphatic massage areas exists.

Time: 60 seconds.

45) THIGH TWIST

Purpose: The Thigh Twist feels terrific. This technique stimulates circulation to the thigh and gives its meridians a twist that helps to improve their energy flow. The meridians involved are those of the liver, kidney, spleen, gall bladder and stomach.

Positioning: Spread the receiver's legs open and straddle the leg opposite to the one you are twisting.

Procedure: Start near the knee and twist your way up the thigh. Place one hand on the inside of the thigh and the other on the outside. As you push away from you and into the thigh with one hand, pull toward you with the other hand. Incorporate a slight twist to the push-and-pull motion. After one area of the thigh has been twisted, move slightly farther up the thigh and repeat the technique, but this time switch hands. Place the hand that was on the inside of the thigh on the outside of the thigh and the hand that was on the outside of the thigh on the inside of the thigh. Also, push with the hand that was pulling and pull with the hand that was pushing. By switching hands and by alternating the push and pull, you can provide the thigh with a better twist. Use the heel of your hand along with the full hand to apply the push so as to achieve more strength and a better twist with less effort. Work slowly.

Repetition: Repeat twice because it feels oh so good!

Time: 30 seconds for both legs.

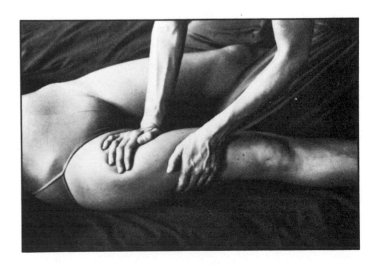

46) PUBIC LYMPH DRAINAGE

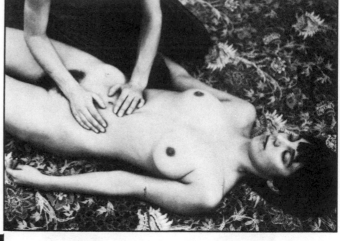

Purpose: This technique forces the lymph fluid of the groin area into the chest where it can be eliminated. It also stimulates sexual function and desire.

Positioning: Sit, Japanese style, between the receiver's legs.

Procedure: Use the full open palm to stroke gently the area on either side of the pubic bone. Move in an upward motion with the strokes.

Repetition: Stroke both areas in unison 5 times.

Time: 10 seconds.

caution, the receiver will jump with a start. Once your hands are gently resting on the receiver's abdomen, you are ready to begin the technique. Keeping your hands on the abdomen, begin a clockwise circular motion. Move from the lower right side of the abdomen up, across and down the left side of the abdomen. Use two hands, one after the other following the direction of movement of feces.

Repetition: Repeat three to five times.

Time: 10 seconds.

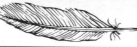

THE TORSO

47) ABDOMINAL/COLON MASSAGE

Purpose: This technique helps to relieve constipation and brings fresh blood to the abdominal area. The internal organs thus receive fresh blood and nutrients to help improve their functioning.

Positioning: Sit, Japanese style, at the receiver's waist. The side of your leg should be touching the receiver's body. Do not lean into the receiver as you work, as your body weight will become very heavy and uncomfortable.

Procedure: Sit at the receiver's side. *Gently* lay both hands on the abdomen with extreme tenderness, for this part of the body is especially vulnerable. Unless you proceed with the utmost

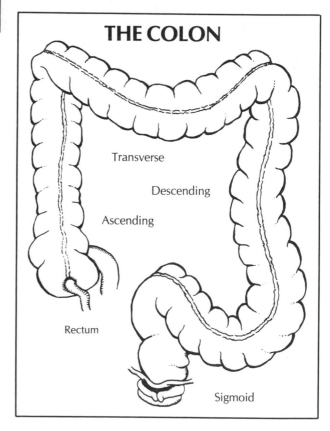

THE COLON

Transverse

Descending

Ascending

Rectum

Sigmoid

48) BOWEL STIMULATION

Purpose: This technique stimulates the peristaltic motion of the large intestine.
Positioning: Sit, Japanese style, at the receiver's side.
Procedure: Begin at the lower right side of the abdomen. Lay your right hand gently over the abdomen and gradually increase its application of pressure. A light to medium pressure is all that is necessary. Next position the four fingers of your left hand between your right thumb and index finger. Gently and slowly insert your fingers into the abdomen. Watch the receiver's face for any grimace that will indicate you are penetrating too deeply. The secret is to penetrate *very* slowly and *very* gently. If the receiver's body senses that you are moving carefully, it will relax and open up to you, and you will not cause discomfort. Repeat the same technique up the right side of the colon, then across the transverse colon and down the descending colon on the left side of the abdomen. When you reach the lower left side, hold the last penetration a little longer than the others. Complete the last penetration by vibrating your hand and arm so that the vibrations extend through your fingers into the receiver's abdomen.
Repetition: No repetition is necessary. If the receiver suffers from chronic constipation, repeat the final penetration and vibration three times. Always apply penetrating force in the direction of the movement of the feces in the bowels.
Time: Hold the penetrations for the ascending, transverse and descending colons for 3 seconds. Hold the final penetration for 5 seconds and vibrate for 5 seconds. Total time: 40 seconds.

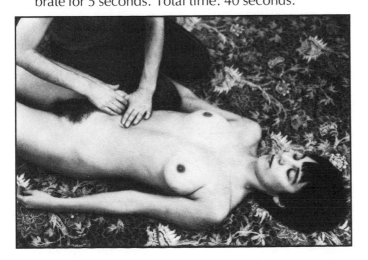

49) WAIST LIFT

Purpose: This technique trims the waistline and stimulates functions of the liver and gall bladder.
Positioning: Straddle the receiver. Your feet should be near the waist and hips. Bend over, but be sure to keep your back correctly aligned. Insert your hands under the arch of the receiver's back.

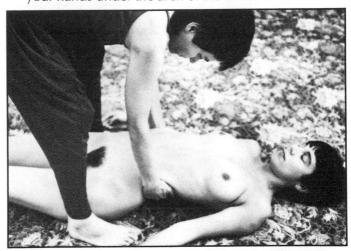

Procedure: Bending over the receiver with your feet on either side of the body and your hands inserted under the arch of the body, lift and pull. Bend your knees as you execute this technique to relieve the strain on your lower back. If you are strong enough, lift the receiver's body partially off the mat. Don't be concerned if you are not. It is sufficient simply to lift the flesh of the waist up off the mat. This technique feels better if executed slowly.
Repetition: Repeat three times.
Time: 15 seconds.

50) LYMPHATIC FINGER FLUSH

Purpose: This technique releases stagnant lymphatic fluids from the lymph nodes located between the ribs. It also aids digestion and stimulates the internal muscles between the ribs.
Positioning: Straddle the receiver with your feet on either side of their waist, or else kneel at receiver's waist.
Procedure: Begin on the side of the rib cage near the waist. Insert your fingers into the intercostal spaces between the ribs. Apply enough pressure

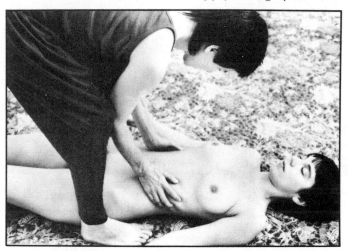

to fit your fingers snugly between the ribs, and continue to apply pressure as you pull the fingers up the side of the body onto the chest. Try to keep the fingers in the intercostal spaces between the ribs, but don't worry if one finger slips out here and there. It's the overall effect that counts. Continue this technique all the way up the chest to the breast.
Repetition: Repeat the technique twice for each area of the ribs.
Time: 15 seconds.

Lungs, Kidney, Heart and Thyroid Neurolymphatic Massage Points are located bilaterally.

51) LIVER & STOMACH LYMPHATIC DRAINAGE

Purpose: This technique improves the functioning of the liver and the stomach. It thus provides an invaluable aid to digestion.
Positioning: Sit, Japanese style, at the receiver's side.
Procedure: Insert your thumbs in the intercostal space between the fifth and sixth ribs on both

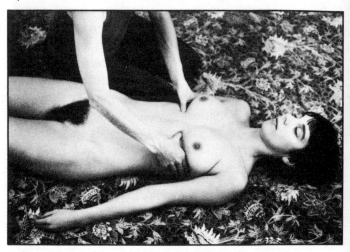

sides of the sternum. Begin near the sternum. Using tiny circular motions, massage the space between the ribs. Locate this intercostal space, which is directly under the breast line in women and directly under the pectoralis major sternal muscle in men, and then massage both sides at the same time. Massage from the sternum to beyond the nipple on the side of the chest.
Repetition: Massage each area of the intercostal space between the fifth and sixth ribs with three circular motions, then move on to the next area between the same ribs.
Time: 15 seconds.

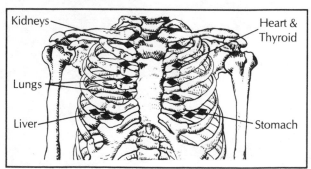

52) LUNG LYMPHATIC DRAINAGE

Purpose: Our lungs have to cope with excessive amounts of pollution and cigarette smoke. This technique helps to relieve the lungs of some of their burden. If you are a smoker, it is wise to massage these points for one minute several times a day.

Positioning: Sit, Japanese style, at the receiver's side.

Procedure: Insert your fingers into intercostal space between the third and fourth ribs, and then the space between the fourth and fifth, on either side of the sternum. Press into these spaces firmly with a tiny, circular massaging motion.

Repetition: Massage the intercostal spaces on both sides at the same time three to five times.

Time: 10 seconds.

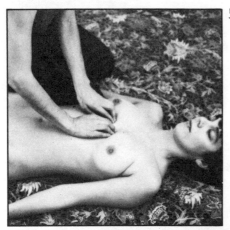
52

53
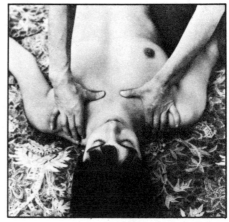

53) HEART & THYROID LYMPHATIC POINTS

Purpose: These points will help improve heart and thyroid functions. Heart problems and thyroid conditions respond to these points if they are massaged regularly.

Positioning: Sit, Japanese style, at the receiver's side.

Procedure: Insert your thumbs in the intercostal space between the second and third ribs on either side of the sternum. Use your thumbs, in a tiny, circular massaging motion. Massage near the sternum only.

Repetition: Massage the area seven times.

Time: 5 seconds.

54) KIDNEY LYMPHATIC DRAINAGE

Purpose: This technique will help improve your kidney functions. It will also help improve kidney disorders when used regularly and frequently.

Positioning: Sit, Japanese style, at the receiver's side.

Procedure: Massage directly over the first rib, which is located directly under the prominent protuberances of the clavicle bones. It is sometimes difficult to locate the first rib. Don't worry about it. Just be sure you are directly under those bony nobs at the base of the neck.

Repetition: Massage the area six or seven times with a circular motion.

Time: 10 seconds.

54

55) BREAST LUMP CHECK

Purpose: A massage is the perfect time to check the breasts for lumps. It should be done regularly, but as many women fear examining their breasts themselves, a breast check once a week during a massage is the next best thing. Early detection has saved many a breast!

Positioning: Sit, Japanese style, next to the receiver.

Procedure: A very light touch is essential. Feel the entire breast for lumps by using a gentle, small circular motion of the fingers. Also inspect the breasts for irregularity of color. Remember that just before, during and sometimes after a menstrual cycle, a woman's breasts tend to be a little lumpy because the glands are swollen. If there is a swelling, and if it does not disappear after the menstrual cycle is completed, it would be wise to visit a homoeopathic doctor. I stress homoeopathy because the herbs used by homoeopathic doctors have saved many a breast that was doomed for removal by orthodox doctors. Surgery should be considered only as a last resort. It is a well-known fact that far too many mastectomy operations are performed each year. Many breasts have been removed unnecessarily.

Repetition: Repeat only when you are uncertain.

Time: 30 seconds.

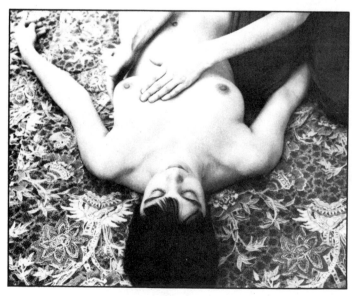

56) SHOULDER KNEADING

Purpose: Tense, raised shoulders respond very well to this technique. Slow kneading helps the shoulders to relax and loosen up. These same points also stimulate brain and lung functions.

Positioning: Kneel next to the receiver's chest and place the heel of your hands into the hollow of the receiver's shoulders.

Procedure: Slowly, but firmly, using your body weight, begin a rocking motion. Alternate your body weight between the right and left shoulders.

Repetition: Rock each shoulder five times, or rock both shoulders a total of ten times.

Time: 10 seconds.

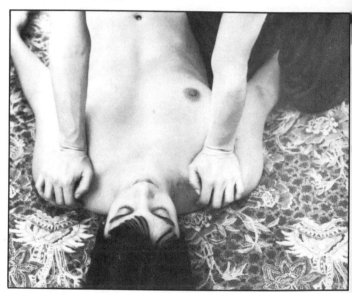

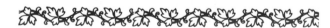

HANDS & ARMS

*Do one hand and arm thoroughly before
doing the other.*

57) HAND FAN SPREAD

Purpose: This technique spreads open the hands to help release stored tension. It also helps to improve the flow of energy along the meridians that terminate in the hand. It thus affects the functioning of the Large Intestine, Small Intestine, Heart, Lung, Heart Constrictor, and Triple Heater/Warmer Meridians, as well as the functioning of the organs related to these meridians.

Positioning: Sit, Japanese style, at the receiver's side below the hand.
Procedure: Spread or fan the receiver's hand. Pull your thumbs first across the back of the hand, then across the palm of the hand. Do not use too much pressure, as it will feel to the receiver like you are splitting or tearing the skin of the hand.
Repetition: Repeat three times on both sides of the hand.
Time: 10 seconds.

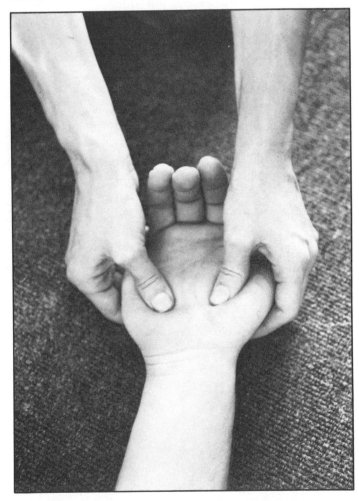

58) FINGER & THUMB MASSAGE

Purpose: This technique returns the blood of the fingers and hands to the heart. It thereby allows fresh blood to enter the fingers and hands. It also serves to stimulate the energy flow of the meridians mentioned in Technique #57.

Positioning: Sit, Japanese style, at the receiver's side.

Procedure: Begin massaging the fingers at the base of the nails. Use your thumb and index finger to apply a firm pressure to either side of the base of the nail. This technique stimulates the flow of energy in the meridian that terminates or begins in the finger you are massaging. Then, with a firm massaging and squeezing motion, move from the tip of the finger to the hand. Support the receiver's hand while massaging the fingers. Twist each finger once in both directions. If you hear a snapping or popping sound, do not be alarmed. This sound is good, for it indicates the finger joints are being released. Next, pull each finger. Repeat the same procedure for each finger and the thumb. Do not massage the other hand until you have completely finished the hand and arm on which you are working.

Repetition: No repetition is necessary.

Time: 50 seconds for each hand.

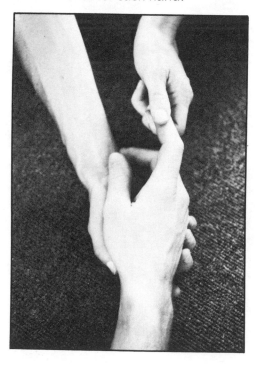

59) WRIST STRETCHES

Purpose: This technique improves the flexibility of the wrist joint, and thus the flow of energy in the meridians that travel along the arm into the hand. See Technique #57.

Positioning: Sit, Japanese style, at the receiver's side below the hand.

Procedure: Hold the receiver's arm with one of your hands. Bend the wrist backward and then forward. Next, bend the wrist to the right and then to the left. Bend gently so as not to harm the receiver.

Repetition: No repetition is necessary.

Time: 15 seconds.

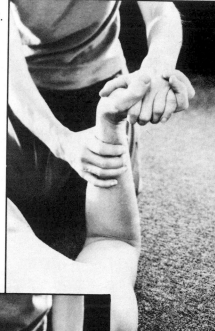

60) FOREARM MASSAGE

Purpose: This is a very general technique, its aim being to force the blood up the arm and back to the heart.

Positioning: Sit, Japanese style, next to the receiver's arm.

Procedure: Begin at the wrist. Massage up the forearm to the elbow with your thumbs on top of the forearm and your fingers on the underside. Use a squeezing and twisting forward motion as you move up from the wrist to the elbow.

Repetition: Repeat twice.

Time: 15 seconds.

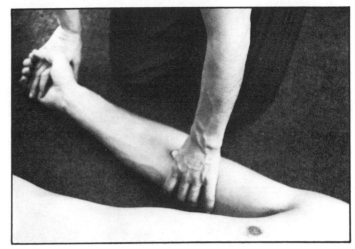

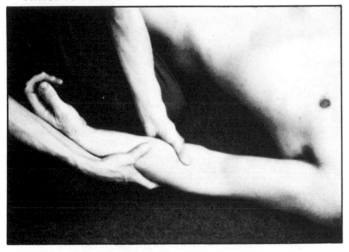

Procedure: Apply a firm, penetrating pressure to the points on all three meridians. Complete all the points of one meridian before proceeding to the next meridian. Use your thumb to apply that pressure. Be sure your posture is correct. See photograph. Your pressure must be perpendicular to the surface of the receiver's forearm so that you will not tire. Apply pressure from the crease of the elbow to the wrist.

Repetition: Hold each pressure point for 3-5 seconds. Use 5-second pressure for those meridians that you feel are most important to the receiver.

Time: 50 seconds.

61) FOREARM: LUNG—HEART CONSTRICTOR (CIRCULATION/SEX ORGANS) —HEART PRESSURE POINTS

Purpose: Pressure applied to the Lung Meridian points helps correct lung disorders. Pressure on the Heart Constrictor points directly affects the receiver's circulation and sex organs, but not the heart itself. The Heart Meridian, which lies next to the Heart Constrictor Meridian, does affect the heart organ.

Positioning: Sit, Japanese style, next to the receiver's arm.

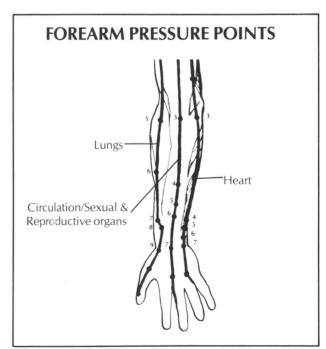

FOREARM PRESSURE POINTS

Lungs

Heart

Circulation/Sexual & Reproductive organs

62) UPPER ARM SQUEEZE & TWIST

Purpose: This technique feels absolutely wonderful, which is the main reason I employ it. Incidentally, it gives the meridians of the upper arm a good twist that enables their energy to flow more freely. It also provides the deltoids and triceps with a nice little massage that helps release some of the tension from these muscles. The meridians involved are the Heart, Lung, Heart Constrictor,

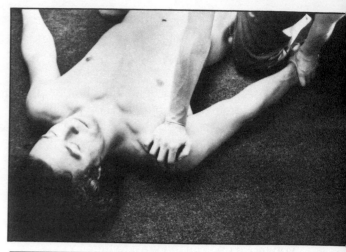

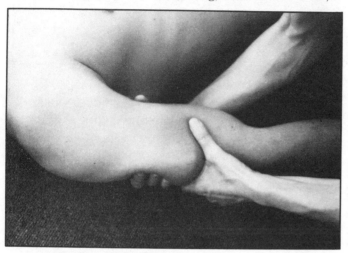

Large and Small Intestines and the Triple Warmer.
Positioning: Straddle the receiver's arm on your knees.
Procedure: Hold the receiver's arm in both your hands. Squeeze and gently knead the arm while twisting it slightly. Continue this technique up the receiver's arm to the shoulder.
Repetition: Squeeze, twist and knead each area of the arm three times.
Time: 10 seconds.

63) UPPER ARM LUNG MERIDIAN PRESSURE

Purpose: This technique improves the flow of energy along the Lung Meridian and helps correct lung disturbances.
Positioning: Execute this technique while you are still straddling the receiver's arm.
Procedure: Use the heel of your hand to apply 3-

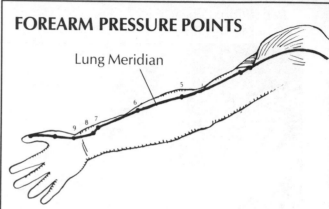

FOREARM PRESSURE POINTS

Lung Meridian

second pressure to the upper arm portion of the lung meridian. Begin on the front of the shoulder and continue down the arm to the elbow.
Repetition: No repetition is necessary.
Time: 10 seconds.

64) TRICEPS MASSAGE

Purpose: Massaging the origin and insertion of the triceps helps to strengthen the muscle, benefits the immune system and helps to regulate abnormal sugar metabolism. The triceps tends to be one of the first muscles to sag. You've all seen people with flabby arms wearing short-sleeve shirts. This muscle can be firmed and toned by regular massaging of its origin and insertion. The origins are located on the posterior shaft of the humerus and along the outside edge of the scapula. The insertion is just below the elbow on the forearm. Each muscle of the body is related to a par-

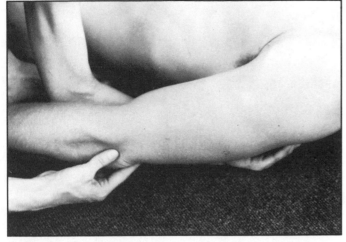

ticular organ, or organs, and is capable of affecting specific body functions. The triceps correspond to the immune system and the spleen as well as the pancreas. Most people, therefore, would benefit from regular massaging of this muscle.

Positioning: Straddle the receiver's arm. Place the fingers of one hand over the top of the humerous near the outside edge of the scapula, and place the fingers of the other hand just below the elbow bone.

Procedure: Use your fingers and a circular, firm massaging motion to thoroughly massage the origin and insertion of this muscle.

Repetition: Massage the origin and insertion of the triceps quite thoroughly.

Time: 10 seconds.

65) ARM TWIST

Purpose: The Arm Twist releases tension from the shoulder and elbow joints.

Positioning: Sit at the receiver's side below the hand.

Procedure: Holding the forearm and upper arm, gently, but firmly twist the entire arm. Twist first to the left and then to the right.

Repetition: A twist in each direction is sufficient.

Time: 5 seconds.

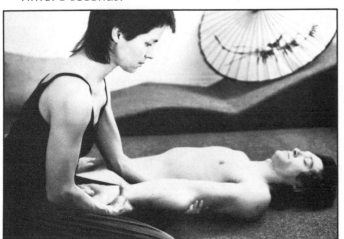

66) CROSS-OVER TECHNIQUE

Purpose: This technique makes the crossing of the body rather simple and unnoticeable. If done correctly, the receiver will not know you have proceeded to the other side of the body. Once there, you will be ready to commence work on the other arm.

Positioning: Kneel between the arm you have just massaged and the receiver's body.

Procedure: Move the receiver's opposite arm away from the body. Place the heels of your hands into the hollows of the receiver's shoulders. Gradually transfer your body weight from your knees to the heels of your hands and your feet. Using your hands as pivotal points, lift first one leg, and then the other, to the opposite side of the receiver's body. The technique is complete when you are on your knees between the receiver's opposite arm and the receiver's body.

Repetition: Unnecessary.

Time: 5 seconds.

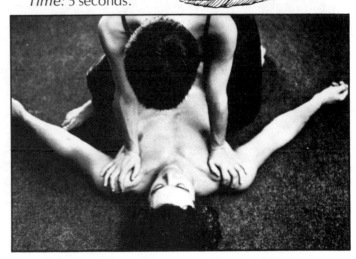

Now that you have completed one arm, repeat techniques #57 through #65 on the other arm.

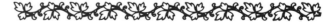

SHOULDERS & NECK

67) ALTERNATING SHOULDER SLIDE

Purpose: This technique helps to release stored shoulder tension.

Positioning: Sit, Japanese style, at the receiver's head.

Procedure: Slowly push one shoulder down toward the receiver's feet. Cup your full hand over the shoulder. Alternate the slow, pushing motion from one shoulder to the other. You must push slowly so that the upper trapezius muscle relaxes. If you shove the shoulder, you will create tension, which is exactly what you do not want to accomplish.

Repetition: Slide each shoulder down toward the feet three times.

Time: 10 seconds.

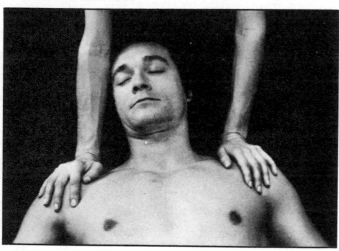

68) SIMULTANEOUS SHOULDER SLIDE

Purpose: This procedure returns both shoulders to their fully relaxed position, releases tension from the shoulder muscles and prepares the shoulders for their position in the next technique, the Upper Trapezius Belly Massage.

Positioning: Sit, Japanese style, at the receiver's head.

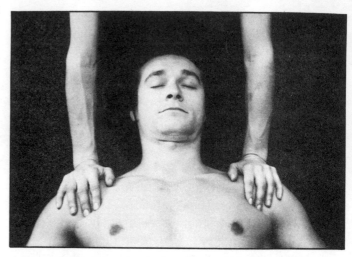

Procedure: Cup both shoulders with your hands, then slowly push the shoulders down toward the receiver's feet. Push both shoulders together.

Repetition: Once is sufficient.

Time: 5 seconds.

69) UPPER TRAPEZIUS BELLY SHOULDER MASSAGE

Purpose: This massage releases tension from the upper trapezius, the major shoulder muscle.

Positioning: Sit, Japanese style, at the receiver's head.

Procedure: Place your fingers under the shoulders and your thumbs on top of the belly of the upper trapezius. Massage and squeeze the entire area. As you do so, incorporate a slight twisting motion. Do not squeeze or massage too hard, for many people will find it too painful. Determine the receiver's tolerance for pain by watching for facial reactions. When you see the receiver begin to grimace, you know you are applying too much force.

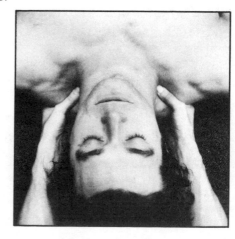

Repetition: Massage the area thoroughly by using approximately twenty-five complete massaging, squeezing and twisting motions. This area needs a lot of manipulation. You will repeat this technique later, after the effects of this manipulation have settled in. When you return to it, you will notice that the area feels looser and less tense, since the previous massaging has released much of the tension from the shoulders.
Time: 30 seconds.

70) SIMULTANEOUS SHOULDER SLIDE

Purpose: Repeat Technique #68. The shoulders tend to rise up from their stretched and relaxed position while you are massaging them. This repetition of the Simultaneous Shoulder Slide returns them to their relaxed position and prepares them for the next technique, Upper Trapezius Thumb Pressure.

71) UPPER TRAPEZIUS THUMB PRESSURE

Purpose: This technique applies firm thumb pressure to the entire length of the shoulders in order to release their tension.
Positioning: Sit, Japanese style, at the receiver's head.
Procedure: Begin applying pressure to the outside edge of the shoulders between the clavicle and spine of the scapula. You will feel a little val-

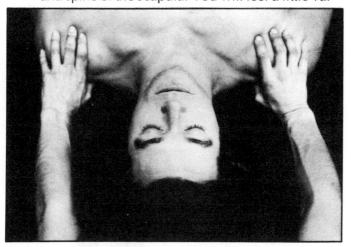

ley with your thumbs, and this is where you begin applying pressure. Move one thumb space at a time as you apply a firm pressure from the outside edge of the shoulders, then along the top of the shoulders and all the way to the neck. Do not skip any area.
Repetition: Apply firm pressure for 3-5 seconds to each area once.
Time: 20 seconds.

72) UPPER THORACIC MASSAGE

Purpose: This technique releases tension from the scapula and shoulder area. Stimulation of the lungs, thyroid and stomach is also accomplished by massaging both sides of the upper thoracic vertebrae.
Positioning: Sit, Japanese style, at the receiver's head.

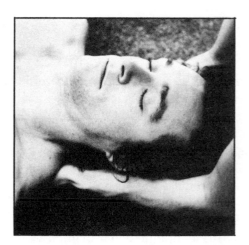

Procedure: Insert the hands, palms up, under the back on either side of the spine. Massage and apply pressure to the back so that it lifts slightly off the mat in a rocking motion. Slide your hands gradually up the length of the spine, massaging alongside the vertebrae, until you reach the base of the neck.
Repetition: Do it five times.
Time: 40 seconds.

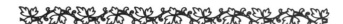

73) UPPER TRAPEZIUS BELLY MASSAGE SHOULDER MASSAGE

Purpose: Repeat Technique #69. Because the shoulders are one of the tensest parts of the body, most people feel neither emotionally nor physically satisfied by only one massage of the belly of the upper trapezius. Repetition of this technique will indicate to you that, although much of the receiver's stored tension has been released, more remains. The repetition will indicate to the receiver your awareness of this lingering pocket of tension, as well as your desire and determination to alleviate it. During this repetition of Technique #69, the receiver usually releases most of the remaining stored shoulder tension. If tense shoulders are a chronic problem with the receiver, repeat Technique #69 again at a later time in the massage.

74) SCAPULA STRETCH

Purpose: The rhomboids muscle originates along the upper thoracic vertebrae and inserts along the vertebral edge of the scapula or shoulder blade. When this muscle is tense, it pulls the scapula out of its proper position. By hooking your fingers along the inside edge of both scapulae and then pulling out and away from the spine, you can help this muscle to relax. You thus help the shoulder blades return to their normal position. This technique will also improve tense shoulders.

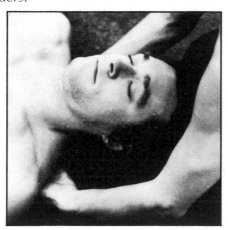

Positioning: Sit, Japanese style, at the receiver's head. Lower your torso sufficiently to execute the technique, but keep your spine erect.
Procedure: Insert both hands, palms up, under the upper back. Hook all four fingers of each hand around the edge of the scapula closest to the spine, then slowly, but firmly pull the scapula out and away from the body.
Repetition: Repeat the pulling motion three times.
Time: 10 seconds.

75) SIMULTANEOUS SHOULDER SLIDE

Purpose: Repeat Technique #68. The execution of Technique #74 tends to cause the shoulders to lose the natural downward position you have helped them to attain. Repetition of the Simultaneous Shoulder Slide returns the shoulders to a relaxed position. It also reminds the receiver where the shoulders should be.

76) SCAPULAE MASSAGE

Purpose: The Scapulae Massage helps to loosen tense shoulders and tense scapulae. It also helps to improve the functioning of the small intestine.
Positioning: Sit, Japanese style, at receiver's head. Lower your torso sufficiently to perform the technique.

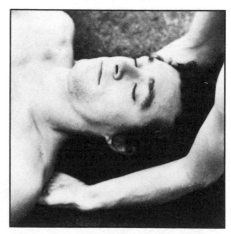

Procedure: Massage the entire surface and edges of the scapulae with four fingers. You need not apply a great deal of pressure because the weight of the receiver's back falling onto your probing fingers will supply sufficient penetration. Use a circular finger massage followed by an inwardly penetrating four-finger pressure to complete the manipulation of each area of the scapulae.

Repetition: Massage each area of the scapulae, then follow with four-finger pressure two or three times.

Time: 20 seconds.

77) NECK STROKING

Purpose: This stroking indicates to the receiver that you are about to begin massaging the neck. As it is incredibly relaxing and pleasurable, many people prefer this simple technique above all others. When correctly executed, it gives the receiver a light-headed sensation and tingling scalp, as well as the feeling that tingles are running up and down the neck, shoulders and spine. Sometimes the tingling will travel all the way to the toes. I interpret these tingles as nerve impulses darting from the cervical region over the entire body because of energy freed and emitted from the neck, a critical point of blockage in the body. These tingles greatly help the body to release much of its stored tension.

Positioning: Sit, Japanese style, at the receiver's head.

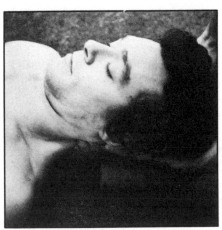

Procedure: Position one hand under the base of the skull and the other under the remainder of the neck. With your hands moving in alternation, employ a pulling motion up from the base of the neck to the back of the skull. Your hands must conform to the contours of the receiver's neck while they are alternately maintaining a good firm grip on the neck and executing an upward pulling motion.

Repetition: Pull hands upward in the Neck Stroking technique at least a total of ten times.

Time: 15 seconds.

78) NECK MASSAGE

Purpose: This technique helps to loosen and relax tense neck muscles.

Positioning: Sit, Japanese style, at the receiver's head.

Procedure: Place one hand, palm down, over the receiver's forehead and the other, palm up, under the neck. Use the fingers and thumb of the hand under the neck to massage and apply pressure to both sides of the entire neck. Reverse hands and repeat. The hand over the forehead remains still.

Repetition: Massage ten times with each hand.

Time: 20 seconds (10 times each hand).

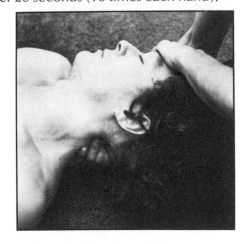

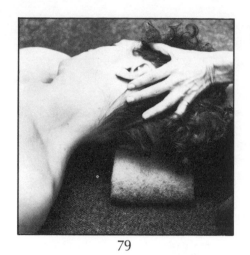 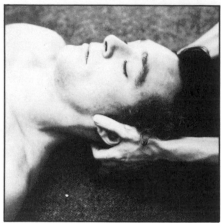 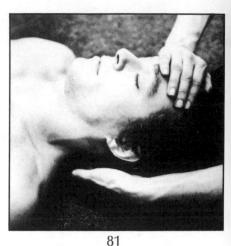

79   80   81

79) HEAD ROLL

Purpose: In addition to relaxing the muscles of the neck and shoulder, this technique helps to release cervical tension.

Positioning: Sit, Japanese style, at the receiver's head.

Procedure: Roll the receiver's head back and forth between your hands. Guide the head to the fullest extent possible in both directions. The receiver must cooperate by allowing the doer to roll the head back and forth freely without any assistance from the receiver. The doer must keep the rolling movement smooth and controlled so that the receiver feels enough trust to let go.

Repetition: Roll head back and forth from right to left a total of five times.

Time: 15 seconds.

80) OUTER PROMINENCES OF THE OCCIPITAL BONE

Purpose: Massaging and applying pressure to the two prominent bulges on either side of the base of the skull releases stored shoulder and neck tension. It is also beneficial to the gall bladder.

Positioning: Sit, Japanese style, at the receiver's head.

Procedure: Place four fingers on each of the prominent bulges at the base of the skull. Alternate a circular massaging motion over and around the prominences with a firm application of four-

finger pressure to the prominences. Pressure must be applied slowly. While applying the pressure, lift the head up slightly and pull it back with your fingers. The head will fall back onto the finger tips, and thus provide a firm pressure as well as a slight stretch of the neck.

Repetition: Alternate three circular massages with one firm application of four-finger pressure a total of three times.

Time: 15 seconds.

81) HOLLOW AT BASE OF SKULL GOVERNING 15-16

Purpose: Massaging and applying pressure to these points helps to relieve neck tension. It is also beneficial to the entire nervous system.

Positioning: Sit, Japanese style, at the receiver's head.

Procedure: Place one hand, palm down, on the receiver's forehead. Use the fingers of the other hand, first to massage and then to apply a firm penetrating pressure to the hollow at the base of the skull. Alternate between these two techniques.

Repetition: When massaging, use a circular motion with three fingers. After completing five circular massages apply a firm penetrating pressure with the same three fingers for 3 seconds. Alternate between massaging and firm pressure a total of three times.

Time: 25 seconds.

82) CERVICAL THUMB PRESSURE FOR NECK TENSION

Purpose: This technique relieves neck tension.
Positioning: Sit, Japanese style, at the receiver's head.
Procedure: Turn the receiver's head to one side and place one hand over the forehead. This hand remains still. With the thumb of your other hand, apply pressure along the side of the vertebrae where the nerves emerge from the spinal column. Begin as close to the base of the skull as possible, and work your way down the cervical vertebrae of the neck. Use a medium pressure. Although firm pressure does the job very well, it is usually too painful. Medium pressure will cause the receiver to feel some pain, but it will be interpreted as good pain and will be tolerated by the receiver because its effects will be felt to be beneficial. When you have completed one side of the neck, turn the head and apply pressure to the opposite side. Switch hands.
Repetition: Apply pressure six times down each side of the cervical vertebrae. Hold each pressure application for 7-10 seconds. Do not repeat this technique as once is usually enough.
Time: 60 seconds for each side of the neck or a total of 2 minutes.

83) NECK STRETCH

Purpose: This technique stretches and relaxes the muscles of the neck.
Positioning: Sit, Japanese style, at the receiver's head.
Procedure: Grasp the head with both hands. Lift it straight up so that the receiver's chin touches the clavicle bones, which are the two bony protrusions at the base of the neck on the front of the body. Repeat the lift, but this time direct the head and chin toward the right and then the left shoulder.
Repetition: Stretch twice in each direction.
Time: 15 seconds.

84) HEAD & NECK PULL

Purpose: This technique relaxes the neck and helps to release tension.
Positioning: Sit, Japanese style, at the receiver's head.
Procedure: Place both hands, palms up, under the base of the skull so that your thumbs are below the ears. Grasp the head firmly and pull it toward you.
Repetition: Repeat twice.
Time: 5 seconds.

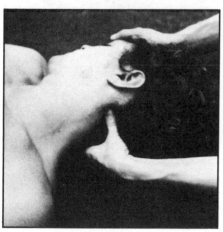

82

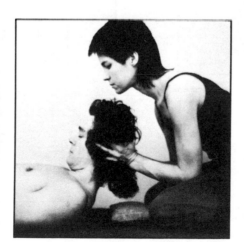

83

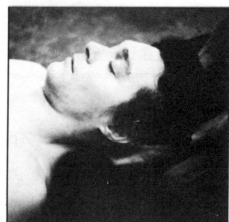

84

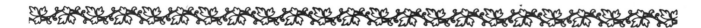

85) NECK SEA WAVES

Purpose: This final technique performed on the neck is another of those particularly marvelous ones. At the same time that it relaxes and releases stress, it provides the sensation to the receiver that her/his head and neck is floating and bobbing on a sea of waves. Everyone loves it.

Positioning: Sit, Japanese style, at the receiver's head.

Procedure: Place both hands, palms up, under the neck. Pull the neck up with both hands and let the head roll freely along with your motions. Trace an imaginary circle in the air while holding the neck. The circle should move in a direction from the receiver toward the doer. The neck is raised off the mat at the highest point of the imaginary circle and touches the mat at the lowest.

Repetition: Make ten circles.

Time: 15 seconds.

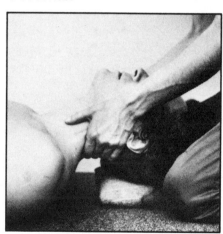

HEAD & EARS

86) FINGER SCRATCH SCALP

Purpose: This technique feels GREAT! It is one of the most popular. The Finger Scratch improves circulation to the scalp, face, eyes and sinuses. It improves, too, the condition of the hair. If employed faithfully several times a day, this technique can also often prompt growth of new hair.

Positioning: Sit, Japanese style, at the receiver's head.

Procedure: Use the tips of your fingers, not your nails. Position your fingers and thumbs behind and to either side of the ears. Using a back-and-forth pulling and sliding motion, scratch the entire scalp. Keep your fingers fairly rigid, and frequently change the direction of your pulling and sliding motion to stimulate the scalp more effectively.

Repetition: Cover each area of the scalp more than once. Keep the scratching motion on the slow side. Although a fast scratch feels good, it will not sustain the receiver's peaceful frame of mind.

Time: 25 seconds.

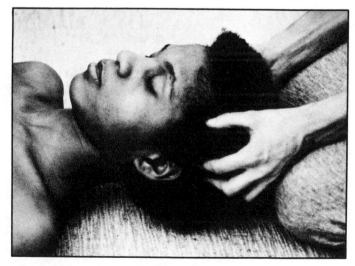

87) GALL BLADDER PRESS

Purpose: This press helps to stimulate and improve gall bladder function. It feels good too.
Positioning: Sit, Japanese style, at the receiver's head.
Procedure: Apply firm pressure to the path of the Gall Bladder Meridian around the ear with your index, third and fourth fingers. See illustration indicating the path the meridian follows around the ear.
Repetition: Repeat twice. Hold each pressure application for 3-5 seconds.
Time: 10 seconds.

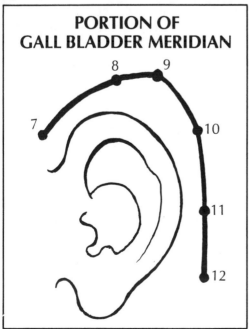

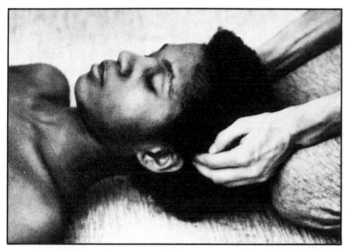

PORTION OF GALL BLADDER MERIDIAN

88) SINUS PRESS

Purpose: This technique relieves congestion and other sinus afflictions.
Positioning: Sit, Japanese style, at the receiver's head.
Procedure: Apply firm thumb pressure from the widow's peak, which is the center of the hairline on the forehead, back along an imaginary center line to the point where the skull drops back. Pressure cannot successfully be applied to the back of the skull from this position.
Repetition: Repeat twice.
Time: 20 seconds.

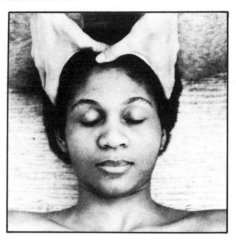

89) FINGER SCRATCH SCALP

Purpose: Repeat Technique #86.

90) GENERAL EAR STIMULATION

Purpose: Stimulation of the entire ear prepares the receiver for the ear massage.
Positioning: Sit, Japanese style, at the receiver's head.
Procedure: Place your index and third fingers on either side of the the receiver's ears. Use a back-and-forth motion and make plenty of contact with the ear.
Repetition: Slide the fingers back and forth a total of five times.
Time: 10 seconds.

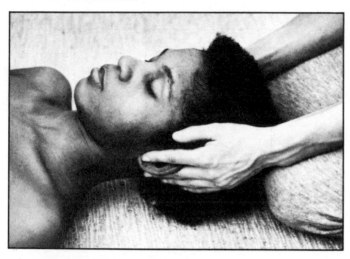

91) EAR MASSAGE

See diagram of Auricular Reflex Points
Purpose: This technique feels marvelous. It also stimulates the reflex points of the ear. Auricular therapy has been practiced in France for many years. Dr. Bordes was the first physician to establish a correlation between auricular reflex points and sciatic nerve problems. Noting that many of his patients with such problems had a scar on the same auricular reflex point, he investigated further and discovered that their local blacksmith had burned the ear at that particular point to relieve their pain.

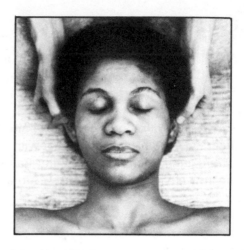

Positioning: Sit, Japanese style, at the receiver's head.
Procedure: Use your fingers and thumbs to massage the entire ear. Do not focus on any one part, but rather massage and manipulate the entire ear.
Repetition: Massage the entire ear twice.
Time: 30 seconds.

92) EAR LOBE PRESSURE

Purpose: Pressure to the ear lobe benefits the face, eyes, sinus and ears.
Positioning: Sit, Japanese style, at the receiver's head.
Procedure: Using your thumbs and index fingers, apply pressure to the entire lobe of the ear.
Repetition: Apply pressure to the entire lobe twice. Hold pressure for 3 seconds.
Time: 10 seconds.

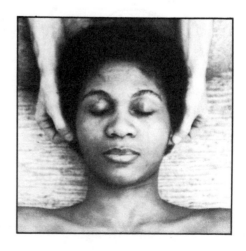

93) MASSAGE & APPLY PRESSURE TO THE EAR

Purpose: This technique is for the further stimulation of ear acupuncture pressure points.
Positioning: Sit, Japanese style, at the receiver's head.
Procedure: Insert your index finger into the eminences and depressions of the ear. Alternate massage and pressure.
Repetition: Repeat twice.
Time: 15 seconds.

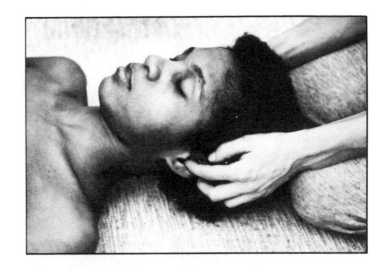

AURICULOTHERAPY

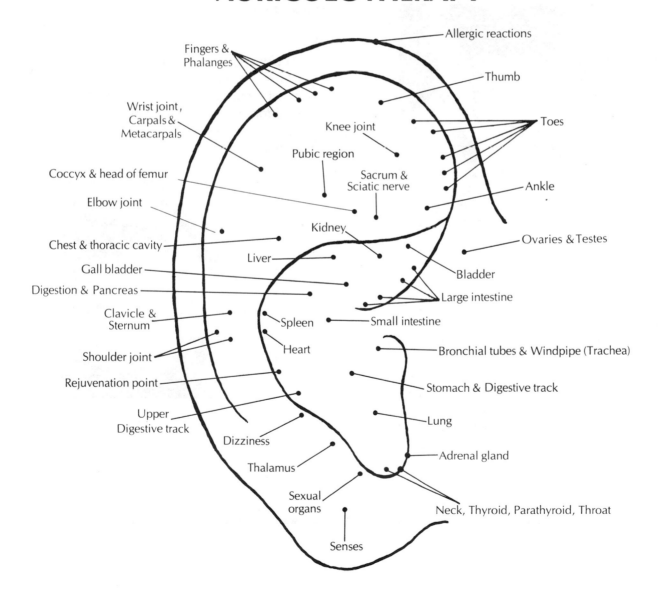

Allergic reactions
Fingers & Phalanges
Thumb
Wrist joint, Carpals & Metacarpals
Knee joint
Toes
Coccyx & head of femur
Pubic region
Sacrum & Sciatic nerve
Ankle
Elbow joint
Chest & thoracic cavity
Kidney
Ovaries & Testes
Liver
Gall bladder
Bladder
Digestion & Pancreas
Large intestine
Clavicle & Sternum
Spleen
Small intestine
Shoulder joint
Heart
Bronchial tubes & Windpipe (Trachea)
Rejuvenation point
Stomach & Digestive track
Upper Digestive track
Lung
Dizziness
Adrenal gland
Thalamus
Sexual organs
Neck, Thyroid, Parathyroid, Throat
Senses

FACE

94) FACE LIFT

Purpose: This technique acts as a greeting to the face. It improves circulation and muscle tone. It also feels really good.
Positioning: Sit, Japanese style, at the receiver's head.
Procedure: Place one hand on either side of the receiver's face. Beginning at the jaw, slide your hands up the face, over the cheekbones and then over the forehead. Allow your hands to conform to the contours of the receiver's face.
Repetition: Repeat twice.
Time: 5 seconds.

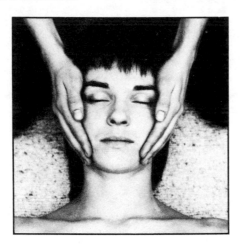

95) CHIN LINE STROKE

Purpose: This technique helps to relax the jaw and trim the chin line.
Positioning: Sit, Japanese style, at the receiver's head.
Procedure: Place your fingers under the chin line and your thumbs above the chin line. Begin at the center of the chin and stroke outward to the jaw. A little oil is helpful for this technique, and the next one too.
Repetition: Repeat three times.
Time: 5 seconds.

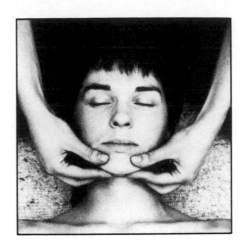

96) CHIN LINE FIRMER

Purpose: This technique helps reduce double or triple chins.
Positioning: Sit, Japanese style, at the receiver's head.
Procedure: Use your middle fingers to stroke under the receiver's chin. Alternate your right with your left hand as you execute the stroking.
Repetition: Stroke each side of the chin under the jaw five times. Repeat more often if the receiver has a double chin.
Time: 10 seconds.

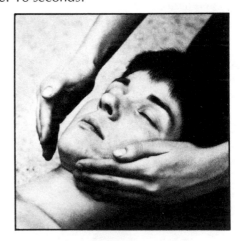

97) GUM PRESSURE

Purpose: This technique helps to improve the circulation to the gums and nerves of the teeth. It also helps firm the lip line.

Positioning: Sit, Japanese style, at the receiver's head.

Procedure: Apply gentle pressure through the skin to the gums of the lower and upper jaw. Use a four-finger pressure technique. Do not press too firmly, for the tissue is sensitive here.

Repetition: One application of pressure to each area of the gums is sufficient.

Time: 5 seconds.

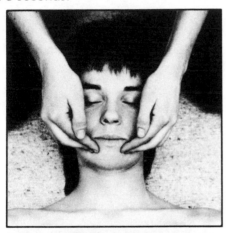

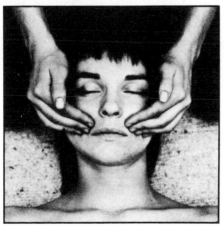

98) MANDIBLE MASSAGE

Purpose: Many people store tension in the muscles of the jaw. This technique helps to release it.

Positioning: Sit, Japanese style, at the receiver's head.

Procedure: Use a circular massaging motion with three fingers over the joints of the jaw. Next, apply a fairly firm pressure for 3 seconds, but be sensitive with your pressure as this is very often a sore spot. Watch the receiver's face for signs of discomfort.

Repetition: Repeat two or three times. Be sure, however, that you have thoroughly massaged the muscles around and over the flexible portion of the jaw, prior to applying firm pressure to the tempromandibular joint.

Time: 30 seconds.

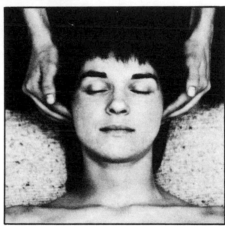

99) CHEEKBONE PRESSURE FOR SINUS PROBLEMS

Purpose: Pressure applied to the cheekbones helps to relieve stuffy sinuses.
Positioning: Sit, Japanese style, at the receiver's head.
Procedure: Use three fingers on the lower part of the cheekbone and your thumbs on the upper part. Apply a firm pressure.
Repetition: Repeat several times if the receiver has chronic or acute sinus problems.
Time: 15 seconds.

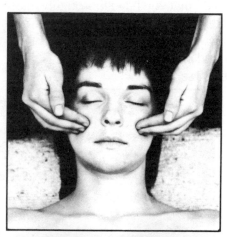

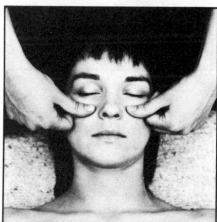

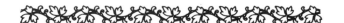

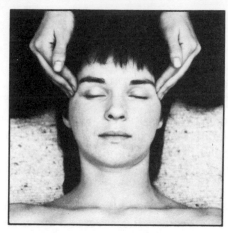

100) TEMPLE MASSAGE

Purpose: This technique is very relaxing and calming. It helps to release facial tension and benefits the eyes.
Positioning: Sit, Japanese style, at the receiver's head.
Procedure: Use three fingers to massage the temples. Begin with a fairly light, circular massaging motion and gradually increase the pressure. Use the pads of your fingers, not your finger tips.
Repetition: Complete ten circular massaging motions.
Time: 10 seconds.

101) FOREHEAD SLIDE

Purpose: Not only does this technique help to relax the muscles of the forehead, but it also helps to discourage vertical and horizontal wrinkles.
Positioning: Sit, Japanese style, at the receiver's head.
Procedure: Position your thumbs between the eyebrows. Slide your thumbs out along the forehead to the hairline just above the ear. Place your thumbs slightly above their previous position between the eyebrows, and then repeat the technique. Continue in this fashion until the entire forehead has been relaxed. Next, use your four fingers to relax the forehead in an upward direction. Begin by placing the fingers of both hands directly above the eyebrows. Gently slide the fingers over the skin until you reach the hairline.
Repetition: The first part of this technique need be done only once. The vertical slide from the eyebrows to the hairline should be repeated two or three times.
Time: 20 seconds.

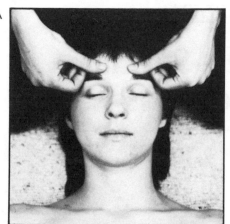
101A

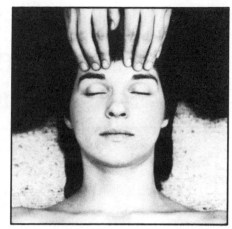
101B

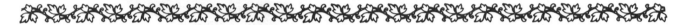

102) ORBIT OF THE EYE PRESSURE FOR SINUS & EYESTRAIN

Purpose: Pressure applied to the orbits of the eyes will improve sinus conditions and decrease eyestrain. Any condition of the eyes will benefit from this technique.
Positioning: Sit, Japanese style, at the receiver's head.
Procedure: Apply pressure to the upper part of the orbits of the eyes with all four fingers. Thumb pressure is more suitable for the lower orbits. Do not be heavy-handed. These points are often tender.
Repetition: Two pressure applications suffice the upper orbits. Apply pressure to the lower orbits as you move from the inner corner to the outer and

hold each application for 3-5 seconds. One application of thumb pressure to each area of the lower orbits is sufficient.
Time: 20 seconds.

103) EYEBALL PRESSURE

Purpose: Pressure here relaxes and strengthens the eyes.
Positioning: Sit, Japanese style, at the receiver's head.
Procedure: Rest all four fingers over the eyeballs and cheekbones. Apply a light to medium pressure. Release the pressure, then slowly slide fingers off the eyes and cheekbones.
Repetition: Unnecessary.
Time: 10 seconds.

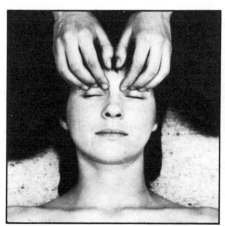
102 A

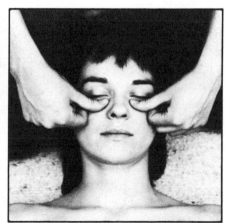
102 B

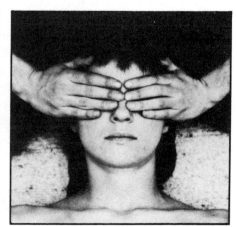
103

CHAPTER V

Massage—Special Applications

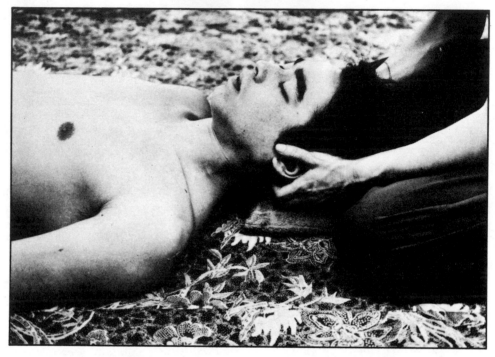

1) "QUICKIE" MASSAGE TECHNIQUES

A Quickie Massage is a wonderful experience. In a minimum of time and with little preparation you can completely change the way your partner or friend feels. Exhaustion, tired eyes, aching back, sore feet, heavy limbs and lack of enthusiasm can be massaged away in a short period of fifteen to twenty-five minutes and can be replaced with renewed energy and freedom from aches and pains due to overwork or worry. An evening or day that might have been spent feeling exhausted, pained and miserable can quickly become a time for fun and new adventures.

Below you will find some helpful suggestions and reminders to make your Quickie Massage a complete success. ENJOY!

- Execute techniques slowly and with great compassion. Quickie Massage does not mean that the techniques are to be executed quickly

- NEVER apply pressure suddenly. Gradual penetration is always the rule

- Try to be conscious of your posture as you massage

- NEVER apply pressure directly to the spinal column

- When twisting, pulling, stretching or flexing any part of the body, always proceed SLOWLY

- Spread a sheet on the floor, dim the lights, silence the phone and begin. Lengthy preparations are unnecessary

Some of the techniques for the Quickie Massage have been extracted from the Complete 60-Minute Body Massage in Chapter IV. Others will be new to you. Those techniques that have already been discussed in the Complete 60-Minute Body Massage are once again illustrated with photographs so that you won't continually have to turn back the pages to refer to the previous section. In the event of any confusion as to what to do or why you are doing it, refer to the more detailed description of the technique in Chapter IV.

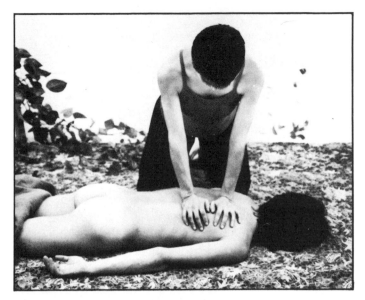

ROCKING THE BACK

This technique prepares the back for deeper penetration and relaxes the muscles near the spine. Sit, Japanese style, perpendicular to the receiver's spine. Use the heels of your hands to rock the back. Rock the upper, middle and lower back five times each. Total time: 60 seconds.

DEEP BREATHING TECHNIQUE

Place the heels of your hands on either side of the upper back. Instruct the receiver to inhale and then exhale. On the exhale, slowly apply a firm, gradually increasing pressure into the back. When you reach the bottom of the rib cage, change the orientation of your hands so that they are perpendicular to the spine and use less pressure so as not to break the floating ribs. The last application of pressure will be directly over the sacrum. Total time: 60 seconds.

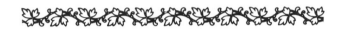

SPINE TRACING

Spine tracing releases superfical spinal tension, relaxes the receiver and prepares the back for the more intense techniques which follow. Sit, Japanese style, next to the receiver. Place three fingers on either side of the spine, then very slowly begin to pull your fingers down the sides of the spinal column. Continue to the tip of the coccyx. Repeat two times. Total time: 20 seconds.

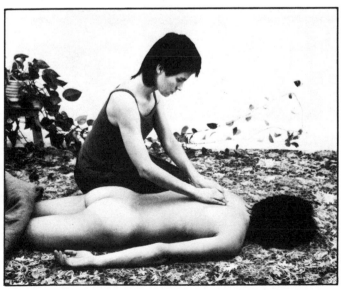

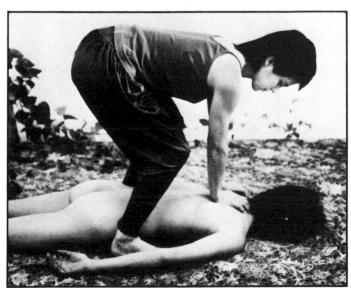

VERTEBRAE TECHNIQUE

Sit at the receiver's side so that you are parallel to the spine, or else straddle the receiver on your knees. In the case of a large person, straddle the body on your feet with your knees bent. Massage 3-5 seconds along side each pair of vertebrae to prepare the receiver for penetration. Penetrate for 5 seconds, then massage 3-5 seconds to soothe. The massaging and penetration should be performed with your thumbs. Place them on either side of the spine close to the vertebrae. Begin midway between the scapula and work your way down the spine to the sacrum.
Total time: 3-5 minutes.

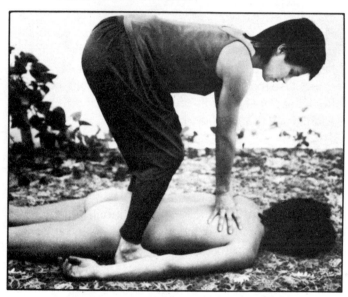

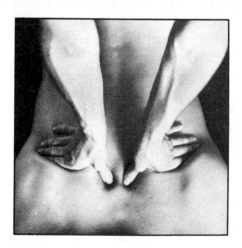

UPPER TRAPEZIUS SHOULDER MASSAGE

Massage, knead and squeeze the muscles between the shoulders and the neck. Use your fingers to loosen and relax the muscles. Follow with firm thumb pressure to any part of the muscle that feels tense or knotted. Total time: 30 seconds.

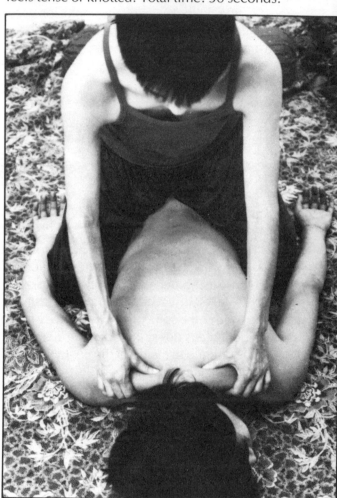

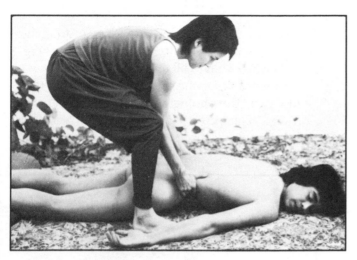

WAIST LIFT

Slide your hands under the receiver's waist and pull the flesh or the entire trunk up off the mat. Apply pressure into the waist as you lift upward. Repeat three times. Total time: 10 seconds.

LATISSIMUS DORSI MASSAGE

Thoroughly massage the fullest part of the muscle by grabbing it in your hands, then knead, twist and release it. Repeat about ten times. As this muscle corresponds to the pancreas, which controls the blood sugar metabolism, massaging it during or immediately after meals aids in digestion. Total time: 10 seconds.

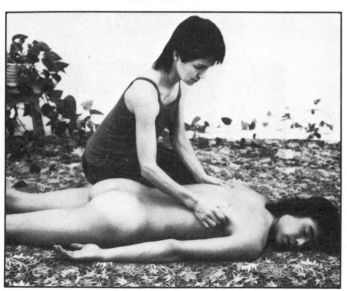

UPPER TRAPEZIUS SHOULDER MASSAGE

Repeat this technique as described previously for an additional 30 seconds.

ARM PRESSURE

With the heels of your hands, simultaneously apply a firm, but sensitive pressure from the top of the arms to the wrists. Use three pressure applications on both the upper arms and forearms. Encourage the arms to roll with each application of pressure.
Total time: 30 seconds.

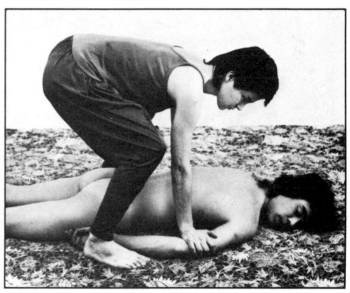

ARM & FINGER STRETCH

Grasp the forearms above the wrists. <u>Slowly</u> pull the arms until the shoulders rise off the mat, then release. Next, massage, twist and pull each pair of fingers simultaneously. Begin with the little fingers and move toward the thumbs. Don't be rough. Pull and twist slowly, compassionately. This technique loosens the joints of the upper appendages and affects all the meridians of the arms which include the Heart, Circulation/Sex, Lungs, Large Intestines, Small Intestine and Triple Warmer. Total time: 30 seconds.

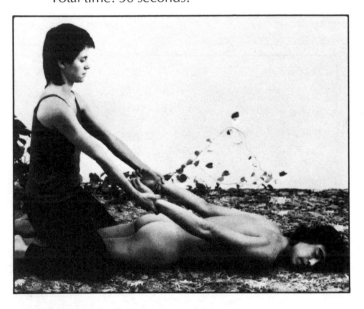

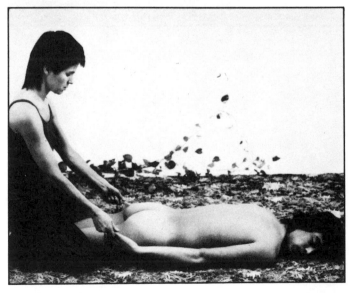

SHOULDER LIFT

Slide your hands under the shoulders. Instruct the receiver not to help but to remain limp, like a rag doll. Slowly begin to lift the shoulders, and then the upper trunk, off the mat. Do not lift suddenly or too high. The photograph indicates how high you should lift the trunk. This technique broadens the chest, relaxes the shoulders and flexes the spine. Total time: 5-10 seconds.

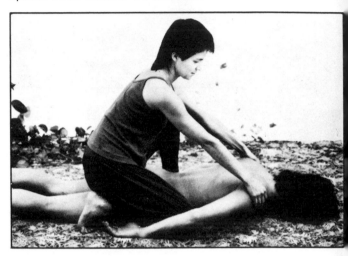

KNEADING THE BUTTOCKS

Knead the buttocks with the heels of your hands. This technique benefits general circulation, the sciatic nerve and the gluteus muscles, which are related to the sexual and reproductive organs. Straddle the receiver's legs and apply a firm kneading pressure. Total time: 20 seconds.

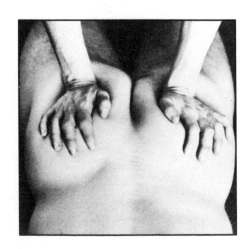

THIGH & LEG BLADDER MERIDIAN

Apply firm pressure for 3-5 seconds with the heel of your hand down the center of the back of the thigh and leg. As the crease of the knee is a very sensitive area of the leg, apply only a very light pressure here. Many people also have tender calf muscles, although they are not usually as tender as the back of the knee. Use less pressure over the calf than over the thigh, but slightly more than that used for the crease of the knee. This technique affects the Bladder Meridian and its associated functions. It also relaxes and releases tension from the leg. Apply pressure to the thigh four times and to the leg four times.
Total time: 30 seconds.

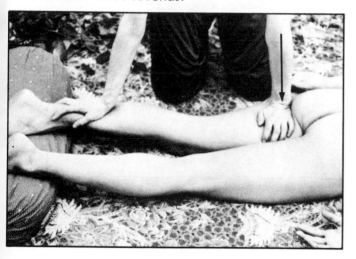

KNEE FLEX

Grasp the feet, bend the legs and *gently* rock them back and forth five times. Next, allow the legs to fall to the side as much as they are able. Rock them in this position five more times. This technique loosens the knee joints and stretches the quadriceps in the front of the thighs. Don't rock vigorously or with too much pressure.
Total time: 10-15 seconds.

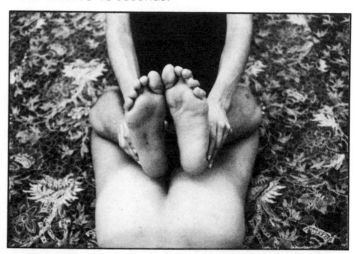

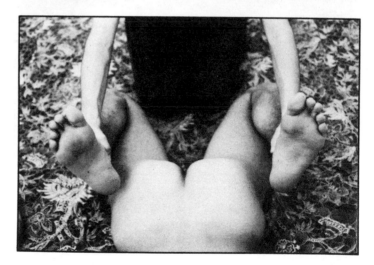

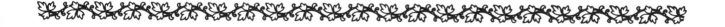

FOOT WALK

With your back turned to the receiver's back, stand on the receiver's feet with your heels. Shift your weight back and forth from one foot to the other. Shift your weight slowly and allow it to gradually bear down on the feet. Beware of the arch of the receiver's foot, as too much pressure on the arch can be painful and could snap the metatarsal bone located directly above the big toe. Before you begin this technique, instruct the receiver to inform you <u>immediately</u> if the pressure is too great. The remainder of the foot can safely tolerate most of your weight for a few seconds. Try to apply pressure to the entire bottom of each foot. Keep in mind the foot diagram and the organs that are affected. Total time: 60 seconds.

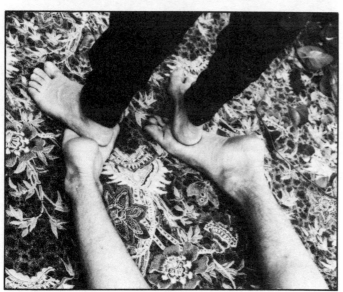

SPINAL SWING

Grasp the feet and *slowly* lift the pelvis off the mat. *Very gently* and *slowly* swing the legs from side to side a total of five times in each direction. Do not lift the thighs more than two or three inches off the mat. This technique increases spinal flexibility. Total time: 10-15 seconds. Do not use this technique if the receiver suffers from extreme low back pain.

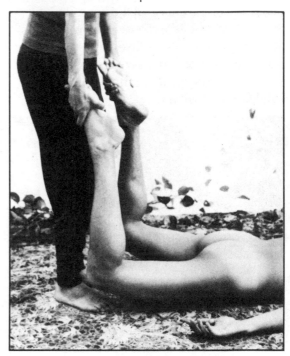

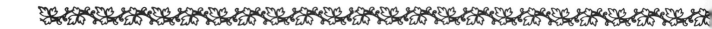

FOOT & TOE ACKNOWLEDGMENT

Because this is a quickie massage and because you have already walked on the receiver's feet, it is not necessary to devote as much time to the feet as you would during a full body massage. Acknowledgment is sufficient to get the blood flowing back to the heart and to stimulate the nerves and internal organs. Squeeze, massage and twist each toe, then apply firm thumb pressure to the arch of the foot and superficially acknowledge the bottom of each foot with your thumb. Complete the foot work with a technique called rolling, i.e. grasp one foot with both hands and twist it in opposite directions from the toes to the ankle. Do not to burn the skin as you twist. Total time: 2 minutes (1 minute for each foot).

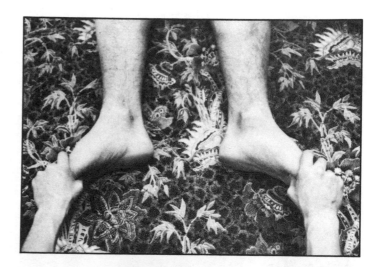

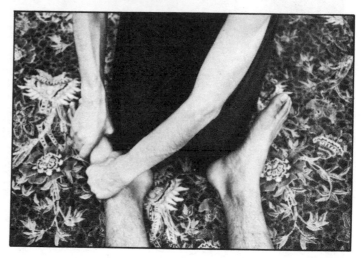

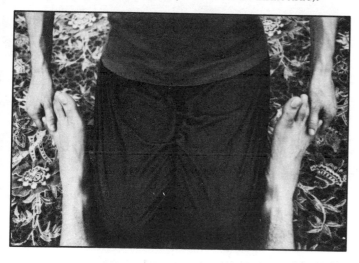

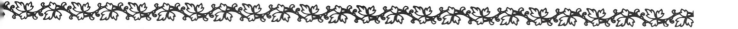

LEG TWIST

Apply pressure to the sides of both feet, first by pressing them outward and then by pushing them in toward the center of the body. This technique loosens the ankle, knee and hip joints. It also feels very good. Push five times each direction. Total time: 10 seconds.

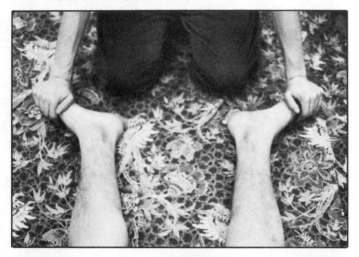

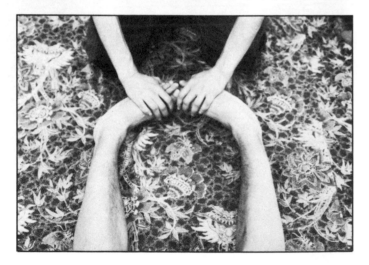

LEG FLEX & ROTATION

Bend the leg at the knee and slowly rotate the leg four times each direction. Encourage the receiver to completely relax so that you can perform the rotations without the receiver's anticipation or assistance. This loosens the joints of the leg. Repeat on the other leg. Total time: 20 seconds.

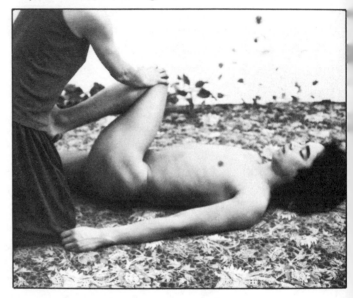

SACRAL PRESSURE

Bend the receiver's legs at the knees. Position the thighs perpendicular to the mat. Cup the knees with your hands and allow some of your body weight to rest directly on top of the knees. Release your weight slowly. Do not apply sudden pressure, as this will not feel good to the receiver. This technique feels wonderful and helps to release lower back tension. Total time: 10 seconds.

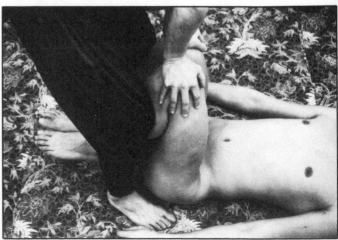

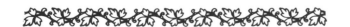

WAIST LIFT

Insert your hands under the receiver's waist and lift up the flesh or lift the trunk off the mat. This technique feels wonderful and stimulates the liver and gall bladder functions. Repeat three times.
Total time: 10 seconds.

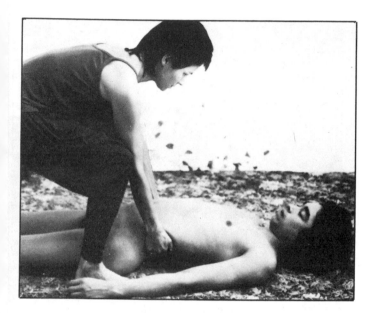

ABDOMINAL MASSAGE

Begin a circular, sweeping motion on the lower right side of the abdomen. Continue upward, across the top of the abdomen and then down the left side. Alternate hands as you sweep around the abdomen. Repeat three times.
Total time: 10 seconds.

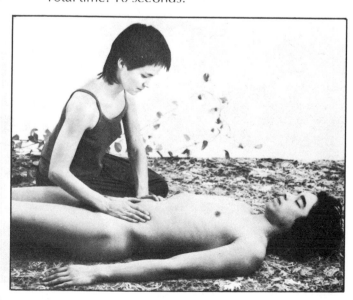

RIB LYMPHATIC FLUSH

Slide your fingers along between the ribs from the side of the torso up to the sternum. Repeat as many times as necessary to insure that most of the intercostal spaces between the ribs have been reached at least twice. This technique feels wonderful and releases stagnant lymph fluid.
Total time: 30 seconds.

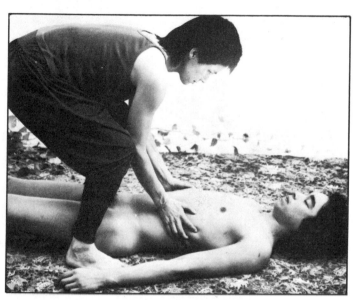

CHEST LYMPHATIC RELEASE

With your thumbs, massage between the ribs on either side of the sternum. Begin under the clavicle protuberances and continue down to the bottom of the breasts or below the pectoralis muscles. This technique benefits the kidneys, heart, thyroid, lungs, stomach and gall bladder.
Total time: 40 seconds.

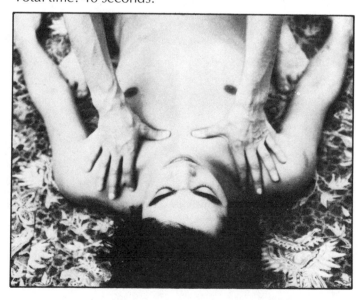

SHOULDER MASSAGE

Insert your hands, palms up, under the upper trapezius muscles. Massage the fullest part of the muscles with your fingers and thumbs. Neck and shoulder tension is released with this technique. Total time: 30 seconds.

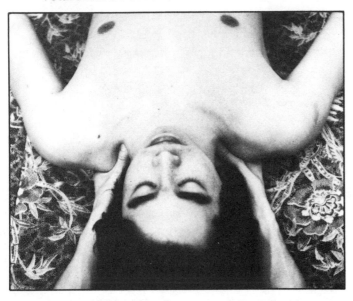

NECK MASSAGE

Hold the receiver's head to one side in one hand and insert your other hand, palm up, under the neck. Massage the nape of the neck with your fingers and thumb. Switch hands and repeat on the opposite side. This technique helps to release neck tension. Total time: 30 seconds.

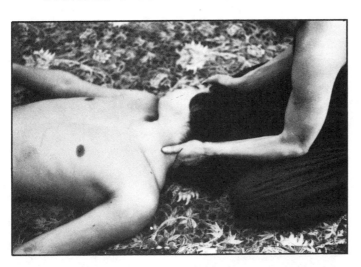

BASE OF THE SKULL MASSAGE

There is a prominent knob on either side of the base of the back of the skull. Position the fingers of each hand over each of the knobs and massage deeply and firmly. This technique releases neck and shoulder tension and stimulates the gall bladder. Total time: 30 seconds.

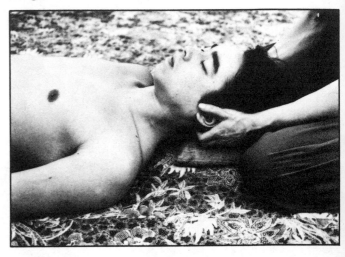

UPPER BACK OR UPPER THORACIC VERTEBRAE TECHNIQUE

Insert your hands, palms up, under the back on either side of the spine. Position your finger tips so that they rest between the shoulder blades, or between the fifth and sixth thoracic vertebrae on either side of the spine. Begin a circular rocking and massaging motion on either side of the vertebrae.

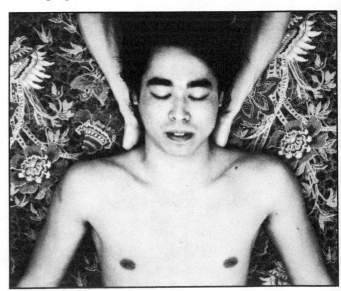

Complete five circular massaging motions, then move up to the fourth and fifth vertebrae and repeat. Continue to the base of the neck. The motion is more difficult to describe than it is to perform. Begin by pushing your finger tips up into the back and then, in a scooping motion toward you, pull your fingers slightly off and back around to same spot. Your finger tips are making a circle that moves toward you and then away from you. At the top of the circle you press your fingers into the receiver's back. Repeat five times between each pair of vertebrae.
Total time: 30 seconds.

SHOULDER BLADE TECHNIQUE

Slide your hands, palms up, under the receiver's shoulder blades. Lift your finger tips up and into the surface of the shoulder blades. Massage each area with circular motions for 3-5 seconds. Then, firmly press your finger tips into the areas you have just massaged and hold the pressure for 3 seconds. Massage and apply pressure to the entire surface of the shoulder blades.
Total time: 60 seconds.

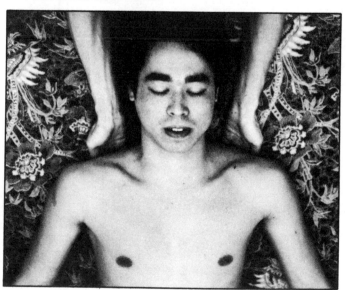

SCALP MASSAGE

Thoroughly massage the entire scalp with your finger tips. Frequently change the direction of your pulling and sliding motions to stimulate the scalp most effectively. Turn the receiver's head to one side when massaging the back of the head, and hold the receiver's forehead with one hand and massage the back of the head with the other. Switch hands and repeat the scalp massage on the other side of the back of the receiver's head. Total time: 30 seconds.

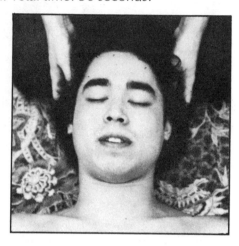

EAR MASSAGE

Use your fingers and thumbs to massage the ears. Go inside as well as behind the ears.
Total time: 30 seconds.

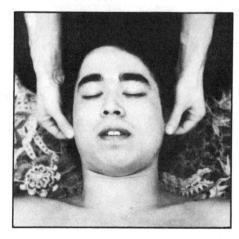

FACE ACKNOWLEDGMENT

There is not enough time to massage the face thoroughly when you are giving a quickie massage. Simply position your hands over the chin and gently slide your hands over the face up into the hairline. The face does not feel neglected as long as it is acknowledged. Repeat five times. Total time: 30 seconds.

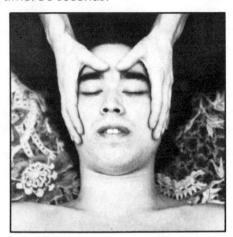

EYE SLIDE

Position your fingers over the receiver's closed eyes and allow them to rest there, very gently, for 20 seconds. Next, very slowly, slide your fingers off the eyes, out over the temples and into the hair line just above the ears. Be careful not to stretch the skin. Total time: 30 seconds.

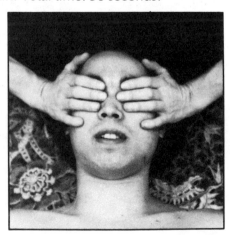

FINISHING TOUCH

Gently rest your finger tips over the eyes and place the palms of your hands over the forehead to make contact with the frontal eminence neurovascular holding points. Remain totally still for approximately 30 seconds while holding your hands in this position. Then, over a period of 20 seconds, very slowly begin to withdraw your hands and fingers from the receiver's eyes and forehead. Once your hands are off the face, continue to withdraw them slowly away from the receiver. A sudden withdrawal is disturbing and tends to startle the receiver, for cool air rushes in where your hands were once providing warmth. Total time: 160 seconds.

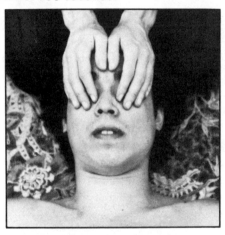

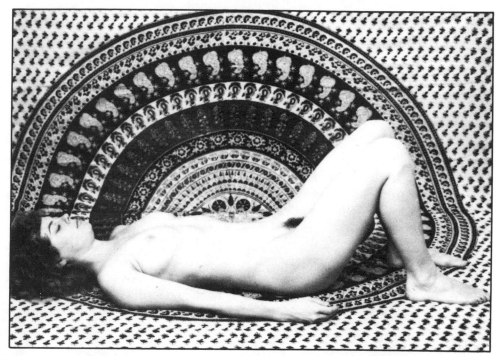

2)HOW TO DO SELF-MASSAGE

Self-massage enables you to care for yourself, both emotionally and physically, on a regular basis. It works, it's simple and it's cheap. No one knows your body better than you. Take advantage of this knowledge by treating yourself to the wonderful sensations and healing powers of self-massage. Granted, massaging yourself is not as fulfilling as being massaged by someone else, but it is much more rewarding, satisfying and effective than most people believe.

People have always touched themselves to relieve pain and release tension. Prehistoric humans no doubt rubbed their abdomens when they were experiencing digestive difficulties and held their foreheads when they were upset or concentrating. Both are extremely common and effective self-massage or self-touch techniques that are utilized on a totally subconscious level of awareness. It's time to acknowledge that our instincts are wise. It is healthy and practical to care for your body and mind. So set aside time once a week, or more often, to improve your health through self-massage.

The method of self-massage taught in this book is unique because it's done exclusively in the reclining position. It thereby eliminates most of the strain and fatigue normally associated with self-massage. The Alexander Rest Position is perfect for self-massage because it minimizes the effort expended. Why fight gravity when it can be used to your advantage?

With legs bent and effortlessly balanced, tilt your pelvis back into the floor (flattening the arch of your lower back) and stretch your entire spine from the coccyx to the base of the skull. Raise your head on a 1"-2" pillow to correct your cervical alignment.

Consider the following while you massage:

* Once you have mastered a technique, focus your concentration more on how the technique feels than on how to implement it

* Keep your body relaxed; don't tense up

* Don't use muscle power; work from your hara

* Close your eyes as you work for greater realization of the different sensations you are evoking from your body

* Try to duplicate the positions shown in the photographs as they will offer you the maximum comfort and greatest result

THE FEET & LEGS

Complete one foot and leg before proceeding to the other.

ANKLE ROTATIONS

Grasp the ball of your foot. Make three slow rotations clockwise, then three counter-clockwise. Feel the stretch and listen for the cracking as the joint loosens up.

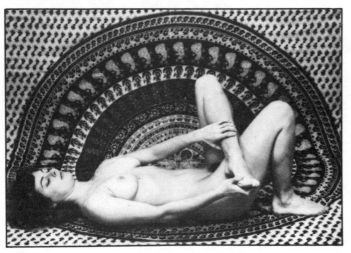

FIVE TOE ROTATIONS

Hold your toes with one hand and stabilize your foot with the other. Rotate all toes three times in each direction.

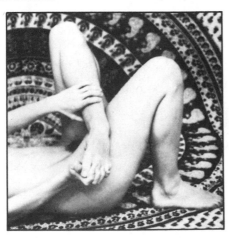

INDIVIDUAL TOE ROTATIONS

Rotate each toe twice in each direction

TOE SQUEEZE

Squeeze and massage each toe from its tip toward the foot. This forces blood back to the heart and out of the toes.

BETWEEN TOE SLIDE

Insert your index finger between each toe. Slide it back and forth three times.

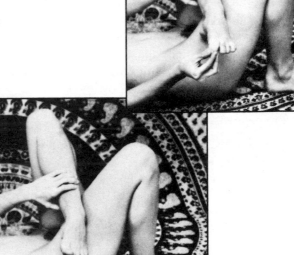

GENERAL SOLE MASSAGE

Use your thumbs to superficially massage the entire bottom of your foot. Circular massaging motions are best to prepare your foot for the more penetrating techniques that follow.

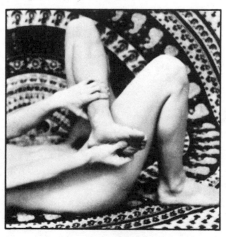

PINCH OUTSIDE EDGE OF FOOT

Use your thumb and index finger to pinch and twist the skin. Begin under the toes and work your way down.

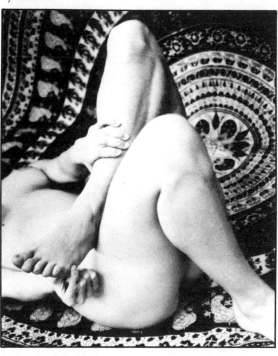

SPINAL COLUMN REFLEX POINTS

Use your thumb or knuckle to apply firm 5-second pressure first to the side of the heel, then up the arch to the top of the big toe.

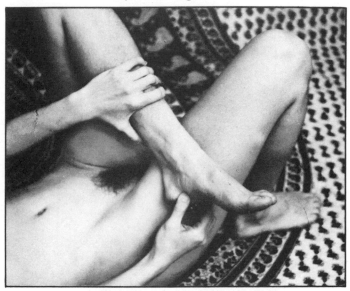

BASE OF THE TOES MASSAGE

Use four fingers to massage the areas under the toes which correspond to the eyes, ears, sinuses and teeth. Press firmly into the bones for 3-5 seconds.

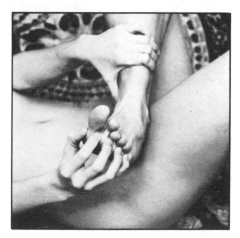

BOTTOMS OF THE FEET REFLEX POINTS

Refer to the foot chart. Apply firm thumb or knuckle pressure to each of the reflex areas for 3-5 seconds. Note that each area corresponds to a particular organ.

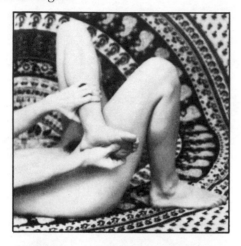

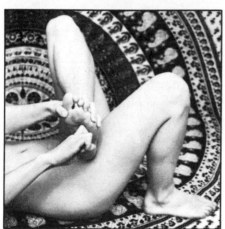

METATARSAL FAN SLIDE

Insert your fingers into the spaces between the metatarsal bones at the base of the toes. Slide your fingers along in the grooves, then up and over the ankle. Repeat three times. This affects the lungs, chest and breast.

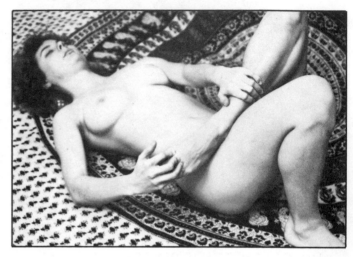

ANKLEBONE MASSAGE

Massage both anklebones of one foot at the same time with your fingers and thumbs. Cup each of the bones with the fingers and thumb of each hand and move them in unison. Use a circular massaging motion. This improves reproductive and sexual organs, hip and sciatic nerve inflamations and back tension.

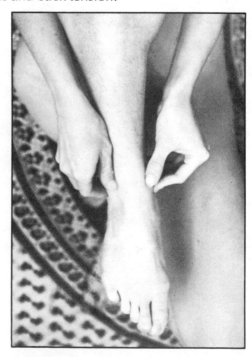

REPRODUCTIVE & SEXUAL ORGANS

Use your thumb and index finger to firmly massage the hollow between the anklebone and heel for 5-10 seconds.

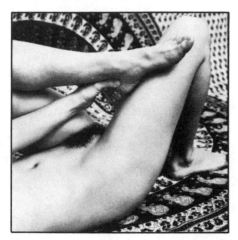

ACHILLES TENDON MASSAGE

Use your thumb and first two fingers to massage and squeeze the Achilles tendon firmly. Sciatic nerve and rectal conditions, as well as disturbances of the reproductive and sexual organs, benefit from frequent utilization of this technique.

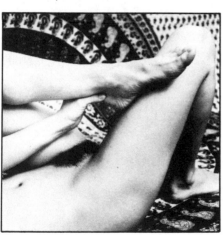

CALF/BLADDER PRESSURE POINTS

Apply a medium to firm pressure to the indicated points with your fingers for 3-5 seconds. Tired legs, bladder problems and sciatic nerve conditions respond to these pressure points.

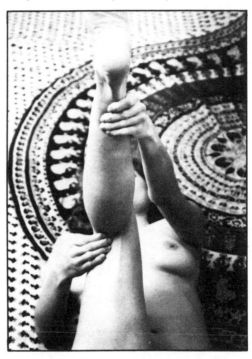

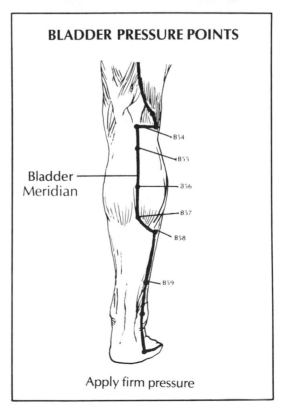

BLADDER PRESSURE POINTS

Bladder Meridian

B54
B55
356
B57
B58
B59

Apply firm pressure

BACK OF THE THIGH BLADDER POINTS

Use four fingers to apply a firm penetrating pressure for 3-5 seconds to the bladder points on the back of the thigh. This technique improves bladder conditions and functions.

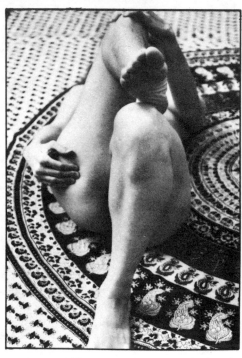

BLADDER PRESSURE POINTS

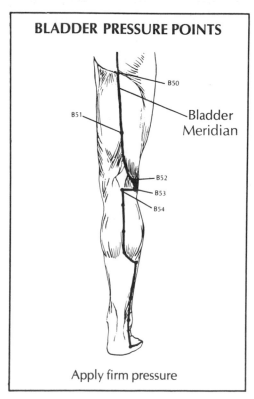

B50

Bladder Meridian

B51

B52
B53
B54

Apply firm pressure

SMALL INTESTINE NEURO-LYMPHATIC MASSAGE POINTS

Use your thumb or your elbow to firmly massage the area shown. These lymphatics not only improve conditions of the intestinal tract but are also extremely useful for low back pain.

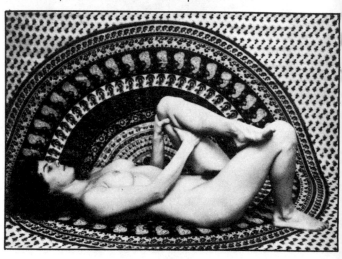

SMALL INTESTINE
Neuro-lymphatic Massage Points

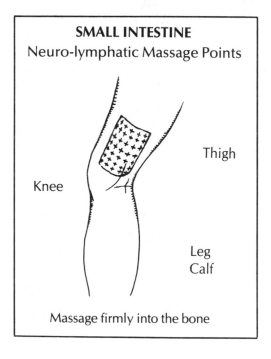

Thigh

Knee

Leg
Calf

Massage firmly into the bone

CONSTIPATION
DIARRHEA LYMPHATICS

Use your knuckles to massage the outside of your thighs. Rub from the knee up to the hip to cure constipation and from the hip down to the knee to cure diarrhea. If your bowel movements are normal, rub up and down to encourage the continuation of normal bowel movements. Reverse recommendation if condition does not improve.

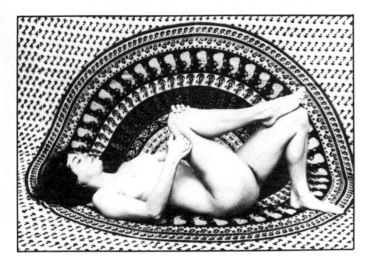

LEG TWIST

Use both hands and twist from below the ankle to the top of the thigh. This technique feels good, releases tension and helps to force stagnant blood and lymph out of the legs back to the heart.

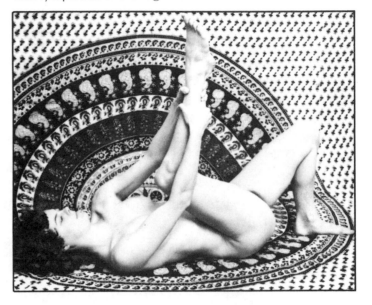

Do the other foot and leg before proceeding to the torso.

LIVER/SPLEEN/KIDNEY
SHINBONE PRESSURE POINT

Use your thumb to apply firm pressure for 3-5 seconds to the indicated point. All the functions of the above organs, as well as infections, respond to this pressure points.

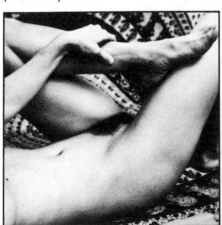

TORSO

ABDOMINAL MASSAGE

Begin a circular, sweeping massaging motion on the lower right side of the abdomen. Continue the motion up and across and then down to the lower left side of the abdomen. It is important to massage from right to left because the feces move in this direction. Repeat the circular massaging six times. Next, apply a firm penetrating pressure with four fingers into the abdomen. Begin at the lower right side and apply firm pressure every two inches. Always press in the direction of the fecal movement. When you reach the lower left side of the abdomen, vibrate and hold the last insertion for 10 seconds. This technique encourages healthy bowel movements.

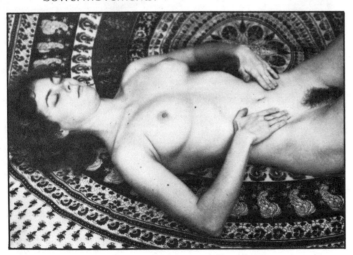

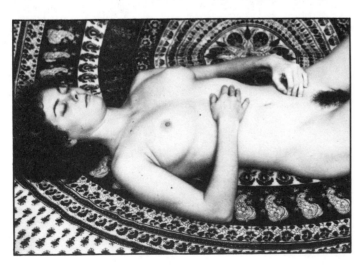

WAIST MASSAGE

This technique helps to trim the waistline and stimulates liver and gall bladder functions. With thumbs forward and fingers back, squeeze and twist the flesh while massaging. Alternate left and right.

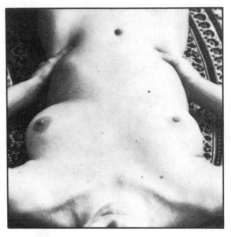

FOUR-FINGER RIB MASSAGE

Begin at the xiphoid process. Massage into the bottom edge of the rib cage from the xiphoid process to the waist and the lower back. Repeat, but this time gently massage under the rib cage to reach some of the internal organs. The functions of the liver, gall bladder, stomach, pancreas and small intestine can be improved by frequent utilization of this technique.

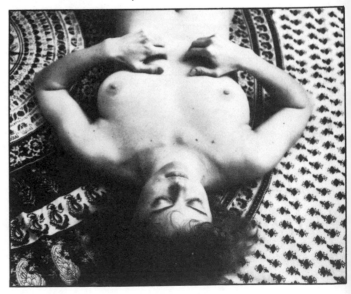

INTERCOSTAL RIB TRACING

Use four fingers and begin in the area of the lower back. Place each finger between two ribs, then press into the intercostal spaces and pull your fingers along, in these spaces, until you reach the sternum. Repeat two or three times, then proceed to trace the upper ribs. Do one side at a time. This technique flushes the lymphatic system and stimulates the intercostal muscles and nerves.

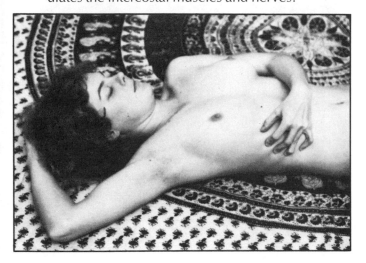

STOMACH/LIVER/ GALL BLADDER LYMPHATICS

Massage for 20-30 seconds, the intercostal spaces between the fifth and sixth ribs. These are located under the breasts or pectoralis muscles, on both the left and right sides of the torso. This improves digestion and disturbances of the digestive tract.

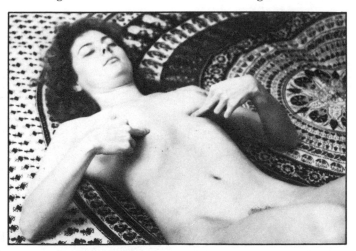

BREAST MASSAGE

Massage in small circular motions and feel for lumps as you do so. Cover both breasts thoroughly.

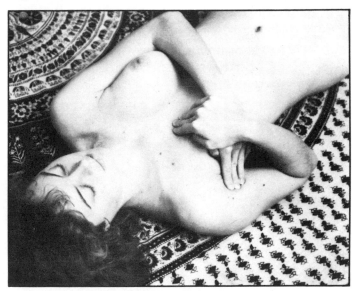

PECTORALIS MASSAGE

Massage for 5-10 seconds the origins and insertions of the pectoralis major clavicular and sternal muscles. This technique not only strengthens and firms the chest muscles but also helps to improve digestion.

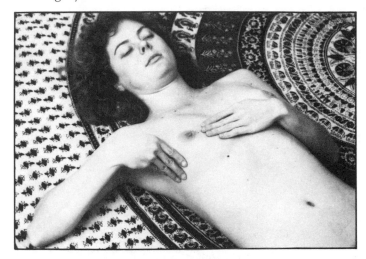

LUNG LYMPHATIC DRAINAGE TECHNIQUE

Massage the intercostal spaces between the third and fourth, then fourth and fifth ribs on both sides of the sternum. These points, which are located directly between the breasts or pectoralis muscles, should be done for 10-15 seconds.

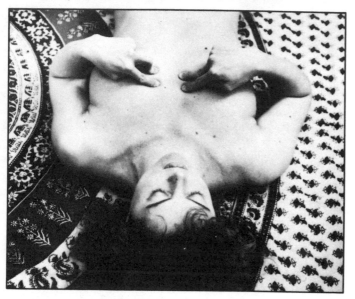

THYROID FUNCTION & HEART

Use your middle fingers to massage between the second and third ribs in the intercostal spaces next to the sternum. These lymphatic massage points help to regulate and normalize heart and thyroid functions.

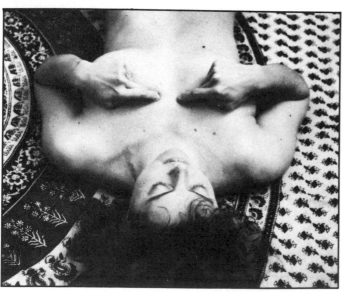

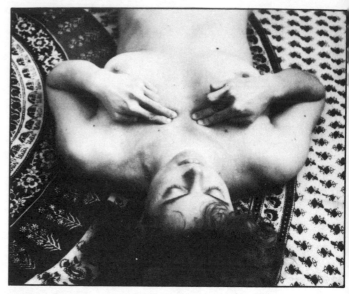

KIDNEY STIMULATION

Massage for 20-30 seconds the first ribs, which are located under the clavicle protuberances, in order to flush the neuro-lymphatic drainage system for the kidneys. Also, drink six to eight glasses of water daily to keep your kidneys functioning properly. Drink before meals or one-and-a-half to two hours after meals. Do not drink while eating as water dilutes your digestive juices.

BRAIN STIMULATION

Use your finger tips to massage thoroughly from the hollow found below the clavicles to the arm pits. Slow learners and people who experience brain fatigue find relief after two or three minutes of massaging these areas. For study purposes it necessary to repeat this technique every few hours, or more often in order to keep the circuits to the brain open and functioning.

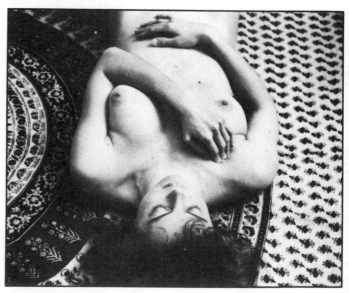

HANDS & ARMS

Massage one hand and arm before proceeding to the other.

FINGERTIP PINCH & TWIST

Grasp the base of each nail between your thumb and index finger. Firmly pinch and twist each finger for 7-10 seconds to stimulate the flow of energy along the meridians that terminate or begin at the nails of the hand.

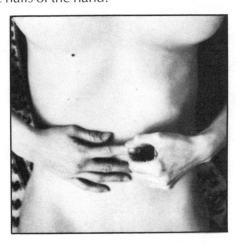

FINGER & THUMB MASSAGE

Massage your digits thoroughly from the tip to the palm. This technique forces stagnant blood back to the heart.

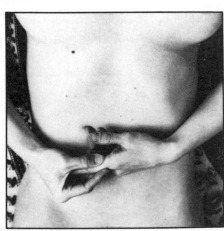

FOUR-FINGER MASSAGE

Position your fingers on the palm immediately below the fingers. Ten circular massaging motions over the bony protuberances in a clockwise direction will stimulate your eyes, ears, sinuses, teeth and brain. Your fingers must be relaxed when executing this technique.

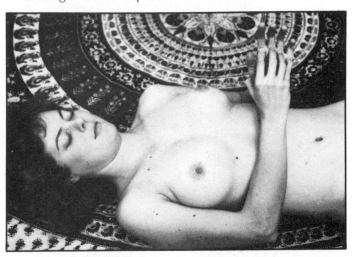

FOUR-FINGER METACARPAL SLIDE

Position your fingers in the grooves directly below the knuckles on the top of your hand. Slide your fingers across the top of your hand and over the wrist. Try to follow the grooves formed by the metacarpal bones. Three upward motions are sufficient to relax the hand and wrist.

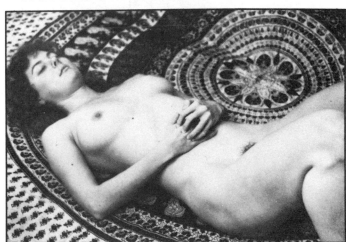

FOREARM ACUPUNCTURE PRESSURE POINTS

Use your thumb to press and hold each of the indicated points for 3-5 seconds. Repeat applications three times if you have a condition associated with these points.

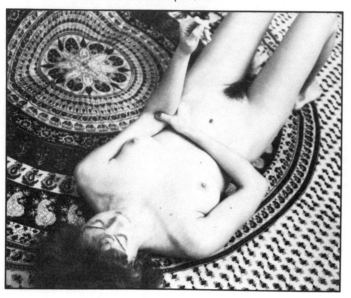

FOREARM PRESSURE POINTS

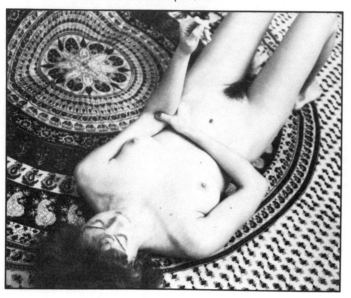

Circulation/Sexual & Reproductive organs

Heart

L5

H3

Lung

C/S3

L6

C/S4

C/S5

C/S6

L7

H4

H5

L8

H6

L9

H7

C/S7

Apply firm pressure

UPPER ARM MASSAGE

Use your entire hand to massage the biceps and triceps. Massage toward the heart and deep into the muscles of the upper arm. Then grasp the deltoid muscles and massage.

Repeat these techniques on the other hand and arm before proceeding to the neck and shoulders.

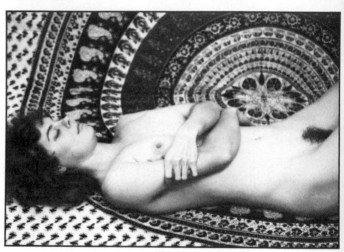

NECK & SHOULDERS

SHOULDER/UPPER TRAPEZIUS TENSION

Do this technique with your arms bent and alongside your chest. Massage the origin, insertion and belly of the upper trapezius muscle with your finger tips. Keep your shoulders relaxed as you massage.

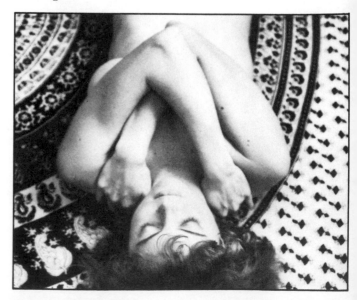

CERVICAL PRESSURE

Begin at the base of the neck. Apply firm pressure to both sides of the cervical vertebrae. Use your middle finger to apply the pressure. Brace it with the fingers on either side of it. Hold each application of pressure for 7-10 seconds.

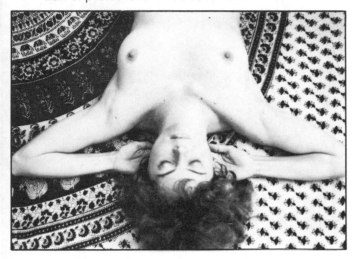

SHOULDER PRESSURE POINTS

Brace your middle finger as above. Beginning at the edge of the shoulder, work your way, with the middle finger, toward the neck and hold each application of pressure for 10 seconds. This technique relieves neck and shoulder tension. Keep your shoulders relaxed as you work.

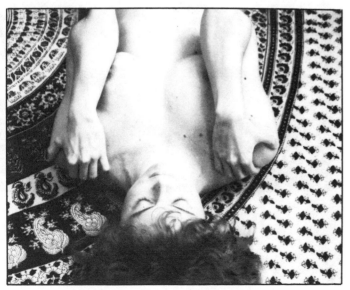

BASE OF THE SKULL PRESSURE POINTS

Use three fingers to apply firm penetrating pressure into the base of the skull. Hold each application of pressure for 10 seconds. Neck and shoulder tension as well as gall bladder conditions will benefit from the regular use of these points.

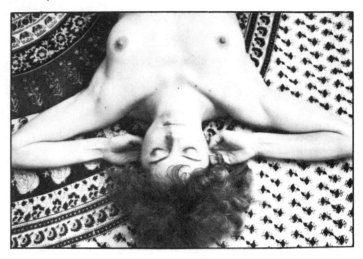

STERNOCLEIDOMASTOID MUSCLES OF THE NECK

Don't let the word throw you. The technique is simple. Use four fingers to massage the large muscle on each side of the neck. Using small circular motions, massage from under the ears to the clavicle protuberances. Do not apply too much pressure as this muscle is usually tender.

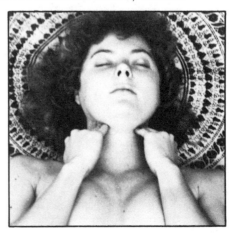

THYROID STIMULATION

Press gently alongside and slightly under the Adam's apple with three fingers for 7-10 seconds. Repeat both sides twice. The thyroid gland produces hormones that keep you looking young.

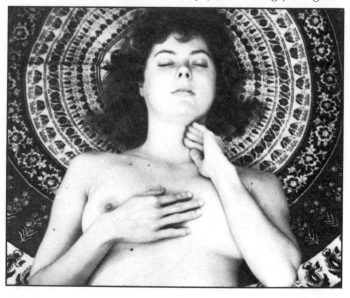

HEAD

SCALP MASSAGE

Using your finger tips or your fingernails, thoroughly massage the scalp. This technique encourages hair growth and improves scalp conditions.

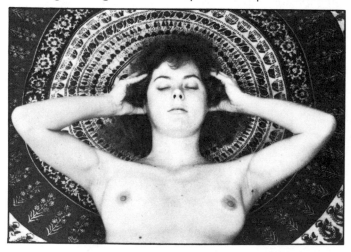

SINUS PRESSURE POINTS

Apply firm pressure with your middle finger as you move from the widow's peak to the top of the back of your head. Hold each application for 3-5 seconds.

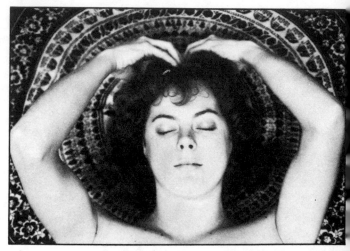

GALL BLADDER PRESSURE POINTS

Apply firm pressure to the Gall Bladder Meridian where it travels around the ear. Hold each pressure application for 3-5 seconds. This technique will benefit the gall bladder and your hearing.

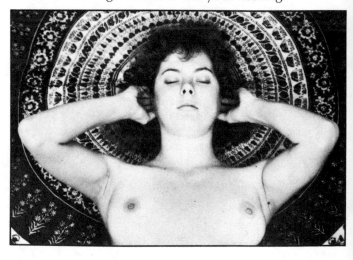

FACE

Use a little cream for the first three techniques.

FOREHEAD STROKE

Slide four fingers from your eyebrows up into the hairline. Repeat two or three times to relax the brow.

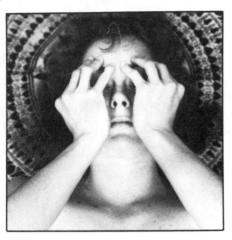

CHEEK MASSAGE

Slide four fingers from the chin up and out to the temples and into the hairline.

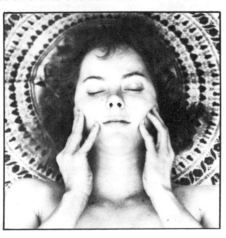

CHIN LINE TRIMMER

With your thumbs under your chin, alternately pull them toward the ears. Repeat two or three times if your chin line is good, ten times if your chin line sags.

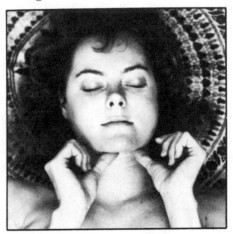

EYE SOCKET—UPPER RIDGE

Apply firm pressure for 3-5 seconds along the entire upper ridge of the eye socket. This technique improves eyesight, relieves eyestrain and benefits sinus conditions.

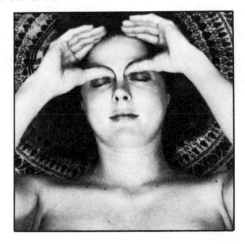

EYE SOCKETS—LOWER RIDGE

Use your index fingers to apply a firm pressure for 3-5 seconds to the entire lower ridge of the eye sockets. This technique yields the same benefits as the upper-ridge technique and also improves digestion.

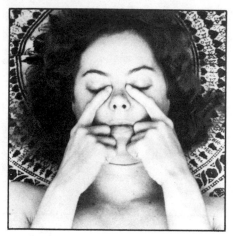

SINUS & LARGE INTESTINE POINTS

Apply a very firm thumb pressure for 3-5 seconds to the entire base of the cheekbones. Sinus as well as intestinal disturbances respond to frequent use of these points.

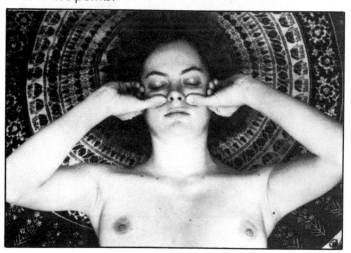

GUM MASSAGE

Use your fingers to massage first the upper and then the lower gums. This technique benefits your gums and the nerves of your teeth. If your gums bleed when you brush your teeth, massage your gums frequently and be sure to obtain additional vitamin C from fresh fruits and natural ascorbic acid supplements. Do not stretch or pull the skin. Lift your fingers off the skin before proceeding to the next area to be massaged.

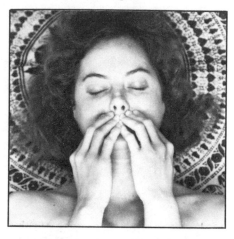

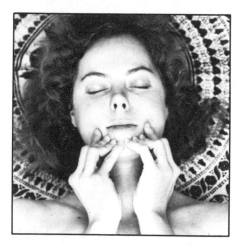

JAW TENSION

Use your thumbs or middle fingers to massage firmly the joints where the mandible meets the skull. Tension accumulates in this joint, but massage does much to relieve it.

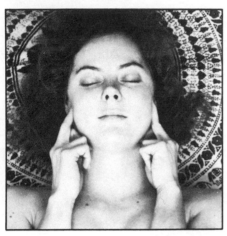

EYE MASK

Position your fingers lightly over your closed eyes for approximately 10 seconds. Do not press into your eyes. Simply rest your fingers lightly on them and allow the heat from your fingers to help relieve eye fatigue. Rub your hands together vigorously to warm your fingers prior to positioning them over your eyes.

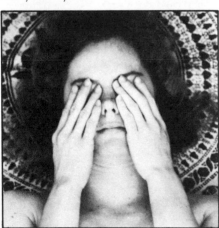

EARS

EAR MASSAGE

There are approximately fifty acupuncture points on each ear. Auricular therapy thus affects the whole body. By massaging, pulling and lightly pinching the ears, you are stimulating the entire body. Auricular therapy traditionally utilizes gold needles to strengthen, silver needles to sēdate and stainless steel needles to balance the body's energies. Ear massage serves the body positively by improving its circulation and energy flow. Massaging the ears also feels wonderful. It may end up being one of your favorite techniques. Begin with the ear lobes, then work your way up and into the ears. Get into all the crevices. Massage, pull and pinch the entire ear. Gently and briefly insert your fingers into the orifice. Hold them there for a few seconds, then vibrate them lightly to stimulate the inner ear.

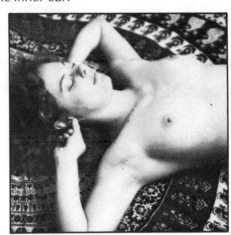

BACK

UPPER THORACIC VERTEBRAE

Use your middle fingers , braced by the fingers on either side of them to apply penetrating pressure to the side of and between the upper thoracic vertebrae. Massage the area where you applied pressure before moving on to the next pair of vertebrae.

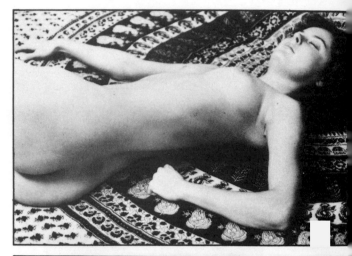

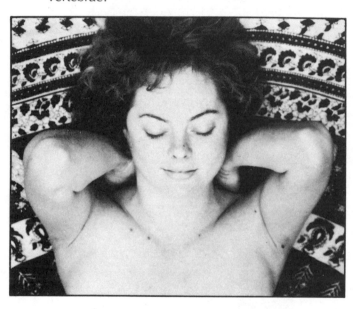

MIDDLE THORACIC VERTEBRAE

Do one side of the spine at a time. Lie on your back with your hip and leg to one side. Form a fist with your hand on the side of your raised hip. Position the most prominent knuckle alongside and between the highest pair of vertebrae you can reach. When the knuckle has been positioned, allow your back to rest on the knuckle. Apply firm pressure for 3-5 seconds, then massage the area with your knuckle. Return to the twisted position and locate the pair of vertebrae just below the one you have just worked. Repeat the technique. Continue in this manner until you reach the eleventh and twelfth thoracic vertebrae.

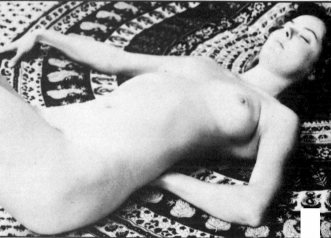

LUMBAR VERTEBRAE

Insert your hands, palms up and with your fingers bent, under your lower back. Use your middle fingers, braced with the fingers on either side of it, to apply firm pressure and then massage along the spine and between the vertebrae.

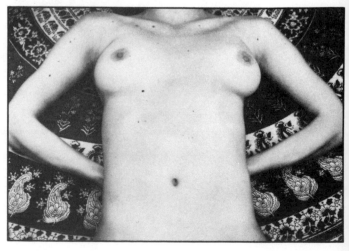

3) A MASSAGE PROGRAM FOR CHILDREN

It's natural for infants to touch and be touched. If a child is deprived of touch during early infancy, or at any other time in its development, physical as well as psychological disturbances are the result. The first twelve months of human life are critical. Adequate physical contact during the first year is of utmost importance for high levels of intelligence, for the proper functioning of internal organs and for emotional maturity. Give your child the opportunity to develop to her/his fullest potential. Begin massaging your child prenatally and continue through the various stages of deveoment, including puberty and adolescence.

Massaging your child prior to birth may seem a little farfetched at first. When you think about it carefully, however, you'll see that it makes sense because touch and massage enhance the psychic union between the mother and her unborn child. Thus, the bond between them will be strengthened, as will their emotional health and stability.

The following photographs illustrate easily mastered techniques of massaging your child through the abdominal wall. A diagram also indicates what pressure/holding points are useful for encouraging a normal and healthy pregnancy, an easy delivery and ultimately, a vibrant baby.

CIRCULATION/SEX
Neuro-vascular Holding Points

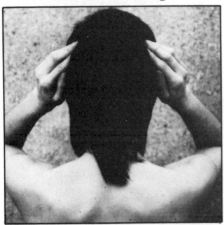

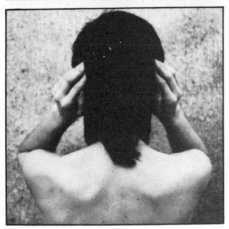

Hold lightly & feel for a pulse

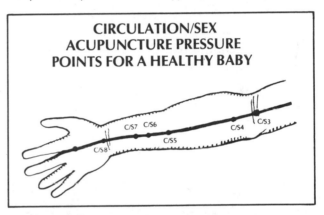

**CIRCULATION/SEX
ACUPUNCTURE PRESSURE
POINTS FOR A HEALTHY BABY**

CLOCKWISE FULL HAND CIRCULAR MASSAGE
Lightly, slowly and sensitively glide your hands in a clockwise movement over the abdomen.

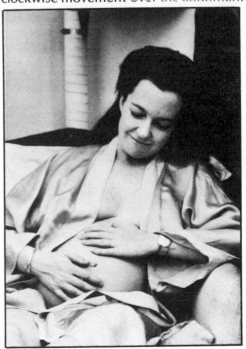

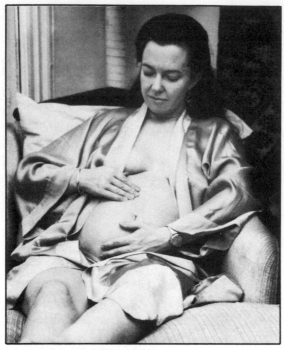

CIRCULAR KNEADING OF ABDOMEN
Stabilize abdomen with one hand and *gently* knead, with slow, small, slightly penetrating circular movements. Switch hands and repeat technique on the other side of abdomen.

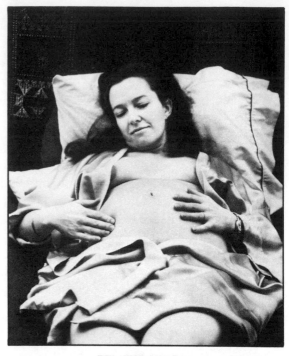

PENETRATION
Use four fingers as one; *slowly* and *gently* penetrate the abdominal wall in numerous places while the other hand is a stabilizer.

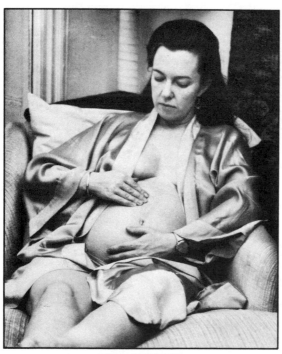

VIBRATIONS
Gently vibrate the abdominal wall in many locations by using four fingers as one.

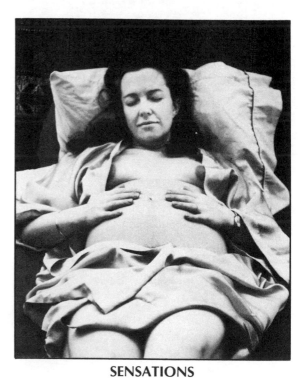

SENSATIONS
Lay your full hands over the abdomen, focus your attention and communicate with your baby. Listen, feel and observe.

Massaging after birth will continue to develop and strengthen the bond between parents and child. It is especially useful to parents who work outside the home, for long daily absences almost inevitably lead to some estrangement of the parents from the child. What better way is there to keep in touch than to massage your child briefly before bed?

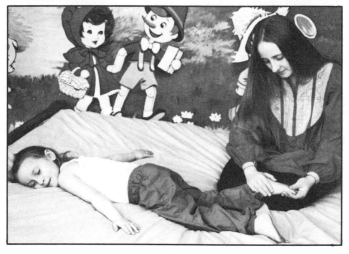

Many children are eager to learn massage and are quite capable of giving one. Encourage your child to massage you on occasion. As young children can easily be overwhelmed by the immensity of an adult body, suggest that your child massage only one part of your body, such as your face, or perhaps one hand or foot. Massage is a highly effective method of strengthening and maintaining the love, trust and compassion between you and your child.

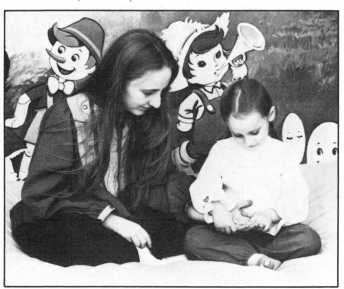

Massage for children can be approached in several different ways. You can set aside one day a week for a Complete 60-Minute Body Massage, you can utilize your favorite techniques frequently throughout the week, you can use specific techniques as they are required, or, you can combine all of the above approaches.

The Complete 60-Minute Body Massage can be readily adapted to a massage routine that is very pleasurable and healthful to children of all ages. The most important thing to remember when massaging a child is that children require less pressure than adults to reap the same benefits from massage. As children are also generally more open to massage than most adults, their young bodies will respond optimally to light or medium pressure. NEVER apply firm pressure. A young child will not understand why you are hurting her or him, and consequently will develop a dislike for massage. If necessary, when you want to relieve a toothache, for example, you can explain to an older child that although a technique may hurt a little, the pain will help the ache to go away. Good pain hurts a little but helps a lot!

Children who are still small enough to rest on your extended legs during a massage should receive the following reordered, altered and somewhat abbreviated version of the Complete 60-Minute Body Massage. Once a child grows too tall or weighs too much to lie comfortably on your legs, you can implement the Complete 60-Minute Body Massage; but rather than using the heel or whole of your hand, use only two or three fingers or a long thumb.

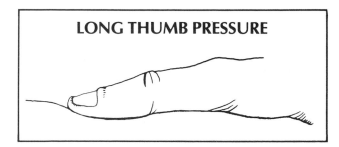

LONG THUMB PRESSURE

You as the doer, can either sit on an armless, straight-back chair with your legs raised and extended on another chair, or else on a bed or on the floor with your legs stretched out. As the ability to move your arms freely is important, place several pillows behind your back. This provides the doer support for the back, which is important as it prevents fatigue and low back pain.

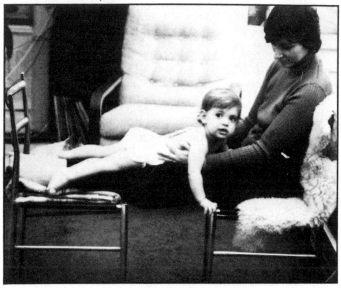

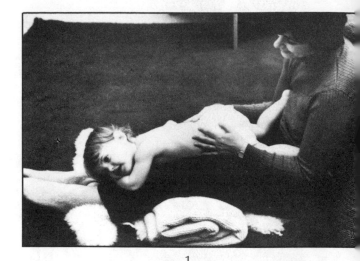

1

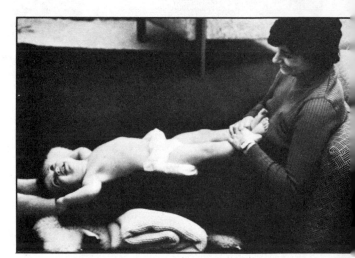

2

The child can be placed in four possible positions. The first is prone (face down) and lying parallel to and on the doer's legs. Be sure either to turn the child's head comfortably to the side or to allow space between and below your legs so the child can breathe easily. Sitting in a chair with your legs raised on another chair assures the child necessary air, but if you feel more comfortable on the floor or on a bed, raise your legs slightly at the thigh and ankle with pillows in order to create the needed air space. The second position is supine (face up) and lying parallel to and on the doer's legs with the child's head towards the doer's feet. In the third position, the child also lies supine and parallel to the doer's legs, but this time the child's head is near the doer's abdomen. Finally, in the fourth position, the child lies prone and perpendicular across the doer's thighs. If you simply cannot work in any of these positions, improvise until you find one that suits both you and your child. Always be concerned, however, with your comfort and the child's ability to breathe.

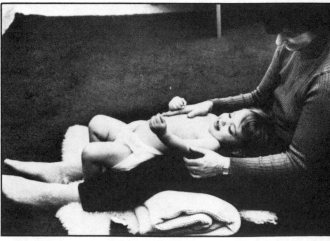

3

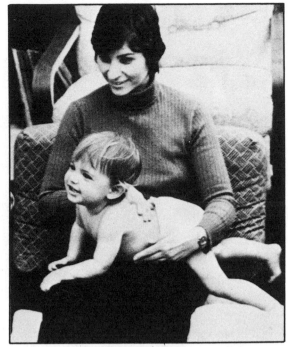

4

Unfortunately, in an attempt to keep the price of this book within range of most people's budgets, I cannot detail each technique as I did in the Complete 60-Minute Body Massage. The following pages, however, have been dotted to indicate a cutting line so that you can, if you choose to, remove them and have them readily accessible when using the Complete 60-Minute Body Massage as your guide.

When referring to the Complete 60-Minute Body Massage while massaging your child, concern yourself primarily with the *Technique* sections. Be certain to use only light pressure and gentle kneading on children. *Purpose* may or may not concern you, for you may be using the techniques simply to make the child feel good. As for *Repetition*, let your instincts dictate how often you repeat a technique. The massage program for small children should be flexible with respect to time. Less than an hour or more than an hour is fine. Finally, *Positioning* is of no importance because your position and that of the child are unique to this massage program for small children.

Do what comes naturally. Touch and massage your child to better physical, intellectual and emotional health. It's never too late to begin. Children of all ages will respond favorably to the introduction of massage into their daily routine.

Section 6 of this chapter provides photographs of the techniques that are useful for common childhood conditions and complaints. Once again, remember that the techniques are always to be performed with light or medium pressure. These pressure points can be used as a preventive measure or as an adjunct to your doctor's suggestions for treatment of the condition.

A MASSAGE PROGRAM FOR CHILDREN WHO ARE STILL SMALL ENOUGH TO LIE ON YOUR EXTENDED LEGS

TECHNIQUE #1: The First Touch consists of picking up, kissing, hugging and then positioning the child on your legs in the supine position with the child's head away from your abdomen.
Then proceed to Technique #31 of the Complete 60-Minute Body Massage.

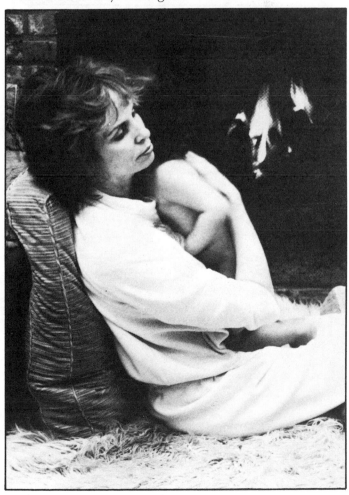

TECHNIQUES #31–39: No changes, but don't forget to repeat Technique #32–37 on the other foot before proceeding to the next technique.

TECHNIQUE #40: Omit.

TECHNIQUES #41–49: No changes, except in Technique #46 use three fingers.

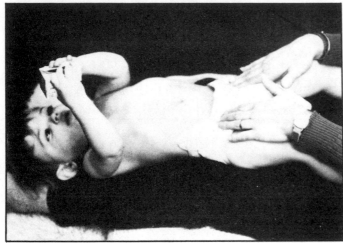

46) PUBIC LYMPH DRAINAGE

TECHNIQUE #50: Omit.

TECHNIQUES #51–54: Use index finger.

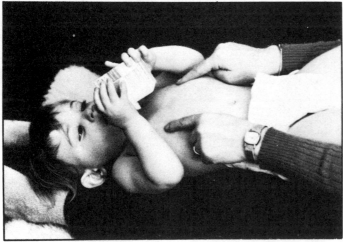

51) LIVER & STOMACH LYMPHATIC DRAINAGE

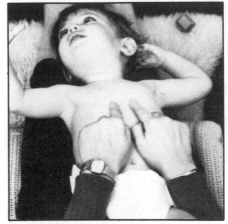

52) LUNG LYMPHATIC DRAINAGE

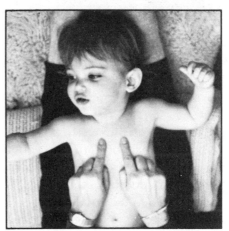

53) HEART & THYROID LYMPHATIC POINTS

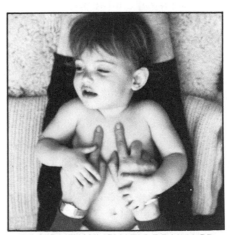

54) KIDNEY LYMPHATIC DRAINAGE

TECHNIQUE #55: Omit.

TECHNIQUES #56–63: No changes, but in Technique #56 use three fingers and in #63 use the long thumb. Don't forget to repeat Techniques #56–63 on the other arm.

TECHNIQUES #64–66: Omit.

TECHNIQUES #67–73: The only change is that of position. Reposition the child supine (face up), with the child's head near your abdomen.

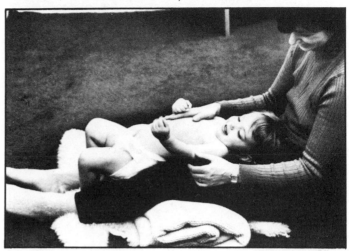

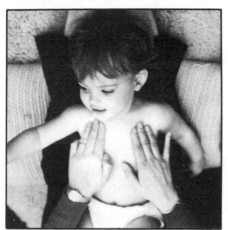

56) SHOULDER KNEADING

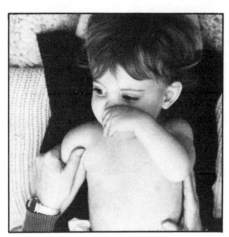

63) UPPER ARM LUNG
MERIDIAN PRESSURE

TECHNIQUE #74: Omit.

TECHNIQUES #75–81: No changes.

TECHNIQUES #82–85: Omit.

TECHNIQUES #86–93: No changes.

TECHNIQUES #94–103: No changes, but in Technique #103 use two fingers.

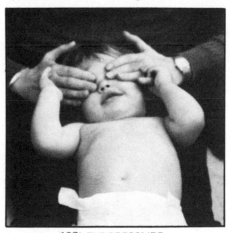

103) EYE PRESSURE

TECHNIQUES #1–2: Omit.

TECHNIQUE #3: Use the index and middle fingers.

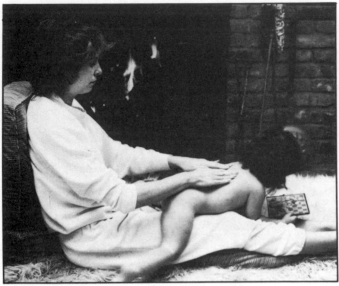

3) SPINE TRACING

Now turn the child over in a prone position for the following techniques. Lay the child perpendicularly across your thighs.

TECHNIQUE #4: Use four fingertips of both hands.

4) ROCKING THE BACK

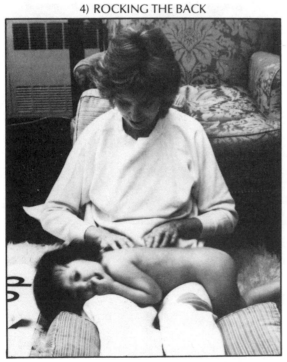

TECHNIQUE #5: Omit.

TECHNIQUES #6–10: Change positioning so that the child is still lying prone (face down), but with the head closer to your knees or ankles. Don't forget to allow for breathing space.

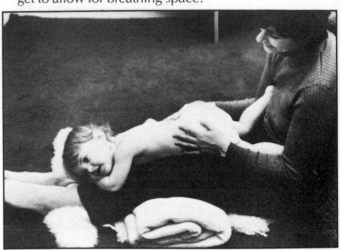

In #6 use your index fingers.

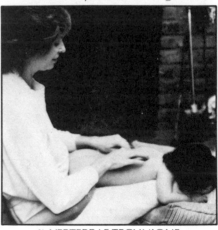

6) VERTEBRAE TECHNIQUE

In #10 use three fingertips together.

10) KNEADING OF THE BUTTOCK

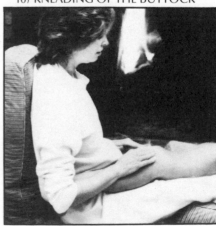

TECHNIQUES #11–14: No change, except in #11 and #13 use the full thumb.

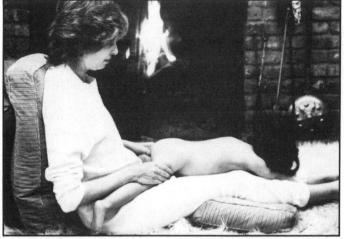

11) THIGH BLADDER MERIDIAN PRESSURE

#26–27 require no change.
#28 should be executed with two or three fingers.

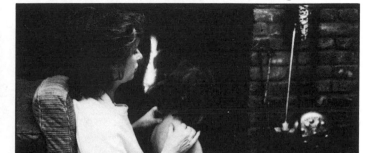

28) SHOULDER KNEADING

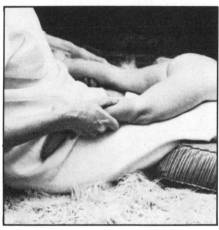

13) LOWER BACK OF THE LEG
BLADDER MERIDIAN PRESSURE

TECHNIQUES #15–21: No changes.

TECHNIQUES #22–30: #22–24 no change.
#25 should be executed with the index fingers.

25) UPPER THORACIC VERTEBRAE TECHNIQUE

#30 implements movements upward from the coccyx to the head.

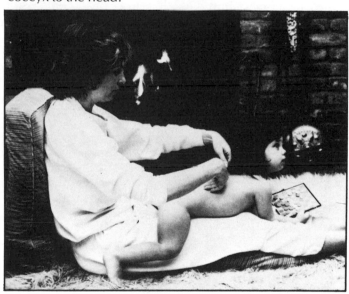

30) FEATHERING THE SPINE

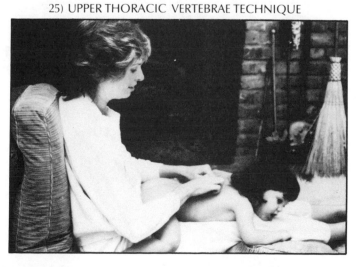

4) HOW TO IMPROVE YOUR PET'S HEALTH & TEMPERAMENT WITH MASSAGE

Animals, like humans, thrive when they are touched or massaged. Animals deprived of touch become withdrawn, aggressive and sickly. If your pet manifests any of these symptoms, you can be sure your pet is in need of massage.

When newly introducing an animal to massage, begin gradually. As soon as you sense your pet has had enough, stop the massage session and wait until the next to proceed with other techniques. Daily mini-massages are ideal between sessions, which can be lengthened as you sense increased willingness from your pet. Most animals will openly welcome massage. There are some pets, however, that have been emotionally damaged. Approach these pets with great compassion and respect. Don't allow yourself to become discouraged if your pet does not respond favorably immediately. Time, love, compassion and massage will eventually resolve most psychological traumas.

Unless your pet willingly submits to massage, begin by massaging a part of the body you know your pet enjoys. After your pet has relaxed and accepts your continued massage of this area, simultaneously begin to massage another area of the body. This technique, or trick, will enable you to get your pet to open up other parts of its body to your touch. Cats or dogs that are aloof or aggressive can be transformed into loving, healthy animals through regular massage.

Consult the drawings depicting the basic anatomy for cats and dogs before beginning a massage so that you will have a feeling for the structures beneath the skin. Always massage the limbs by moving toward the heart in order to return stagnant blood and lymph back to the heart. Never apply heavy pressure, as gentle to medium is usually sufficient.

Below you will find some techniques that I have found to be well-received by pets. Remember, begin by massaging your pet's favorite spots. When your pet is sufficiently relaxed, begin to utilize these techniques.

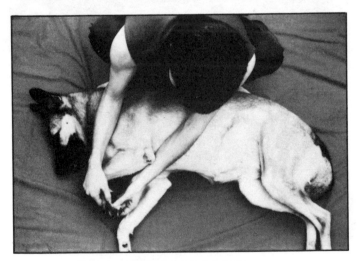

FOOT & PAD MASSAGE

Gently massage the entire foot and then the pads. Massage between the pads as well. The feet are generally quite sensitive, so make your movements slow and easy.

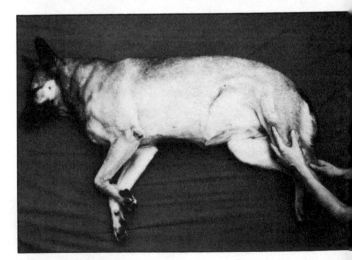

LEG MASSAGE

Begin just above the foot and massage up the leg toward the body. Encourage your pet's leg to remain limp while you massage.

SKELETAL ANATOMY OF A CAT

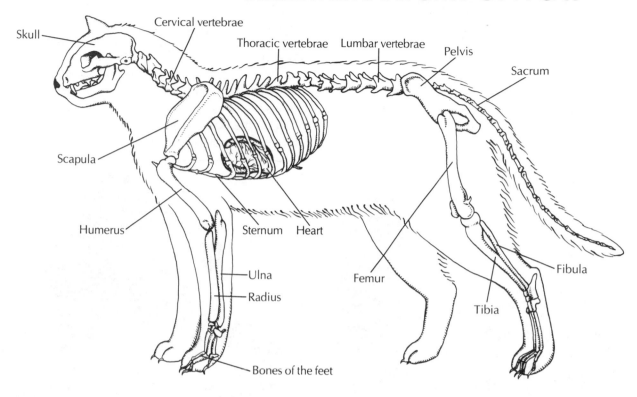

Skull · Cervical vertebrae · Thoracic vertebrae · Lumbar vertebrae · Pelvis · Sacrum · Scapula · Humerus · Sternum · Heart · Femur · Ulna · Radius · Tibia · Fibula · Bones of the feet

SKELETAL ANATOMY OF A DOG

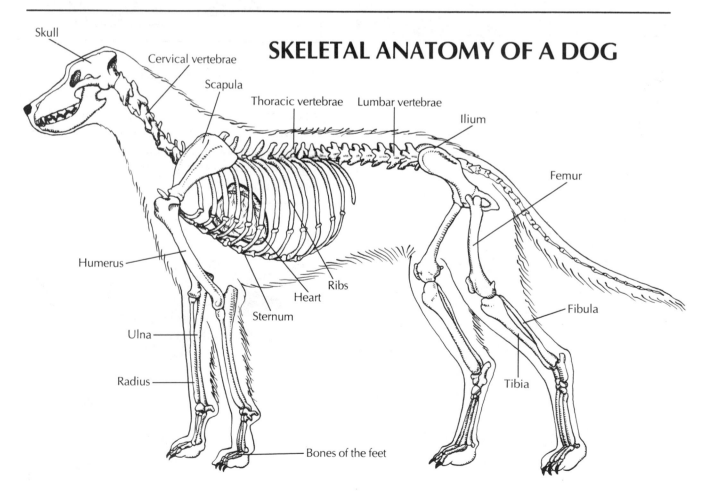

Skull · Cervical vertebrae · Scapula · Thoracic vertebrae · Lumbar vertebrae · Ilium · Femur · Humerus · Ribs · Heart · Sternum · Fibula · Ulna · Radius · Tibia · Bones of the feet

ABDOMINAL MASSAGE

By this time you should have no trouble encouraging your pet to lie spread eagle, but if you do, simply lift one of the hind legs and begin to massage the abdomen. Most pets will expose the abdomen once you begin to massage it. Use two hands, flat on the abdomen, to make circular motions over the abdominal area. With smaller animals, use your fingers as one mass.

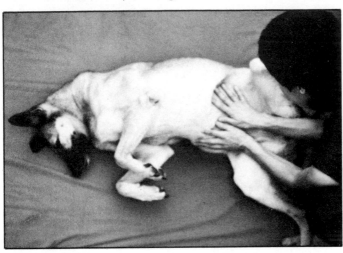

SPINAL MASSAGE

Use your middle and index finger to massage along either side of the spine. Do not massage into the spinal column directly. If you see your dog's or cat's hair bristle or if you see the flesh and hair on the back ripple, you know you have touched a spot that needs attention.

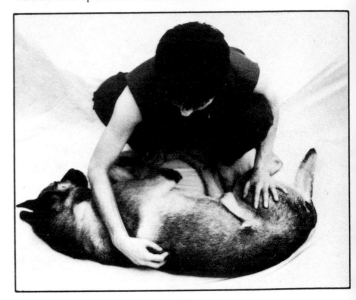

BODY MASSAGE

Massage the entire side of the body available to you. Use large circular massaging motions from the back leg to the neck. Then massage the other side.

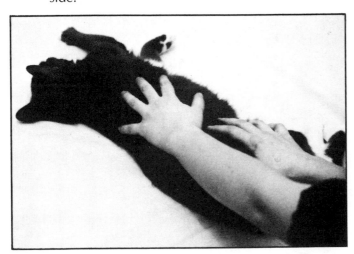

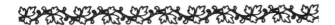

NECK & HEAD & EARS

Massaging this part of the body is favored by most of our hairy friends. Massage thoroughly and linger where your touch makes your pet seem happiest. Massage the neck on either side of the vertebral column as you did for the back. Don't forget the nose or around the eyes.

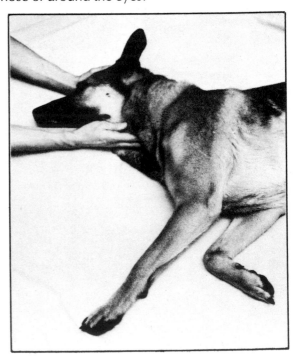

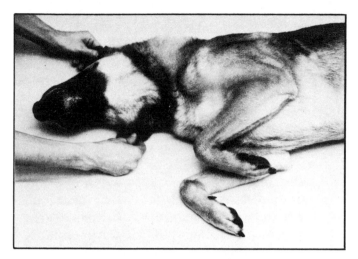

In conjunction with massage, some important dietary changes will better the health and temperament of your cat or dog. Most people feed their pets dry food or canned food. Dry dog food is equivalent to TV dinners. Canned dog food is usually mostly meat, but quite mushy and therefore not good for the teeth. By providing a mixture of moist and dry food, you may think that you can feed your pet properly. I'm afraid not. By introducing the following foods into your pet's diet, you will soon notice an improvement in the way your pet feels and looks. Every pet should have raw eggs twice a week. Dulse seaweed will supply necessary minerals, while salt-free cottage cheese or buttermilk will break the monotony of meat. Dessicated liver tablets and brewer's yeast tablets are treats your pet will LOVE, and fresh carrots, sliced thin, will both clean the teeth and give your pet a slightly sweet treat.

I suggest, too, that you locate a veterinarian who will use herbal remedies or a homoeopathic doctor who will treat your pet if you are under her/his care. Drugs are no better for your pet than they are for you. Try to locate a veterinarian in your area who will work with you and use herbal medicine. Do this when your pet is healthy, however, so that you will know where to get the proper medical attention when you need it.

There are a few books I'd like to recommend to those who would like to treat their pet naturally. The first book listed can be found in many health food stores. The other two are rather difficult to obtain, so I recommend writing directly to the publisher in England. If you are lucky, you may be able to convince your health food store to order them for you. In either case, all three books are well worth ordering and waiting for.

THE COMPLETE HERBAL BOOK FOR THE DOG

by Juliette de Bairacli Levy
Published by ARCO

THE TREATMENT OF DOGS BY HOMOEOPATHY

by K. Sheppard
Published by Health Science Press
Bradford, Holsworth
Devon, England EX22 7AP

THE TREATMENT OF CATS BY HOMOEOPATHY

by K. Sheppard
Published by Health Science Press
Bradford, Holsworthy
Devon, England EX22 7AP

DR. PITCAIRN'S COMPLETE GUIDE TO NATURAL HEALTH FOR DOGS & CATS

by Richard H. Pitcairn, D.V.M., Ph.D.
& Susan Hubble Pitcairn
Published by: Rodale Press, Inc.
33 East Minot St.
Emmaus, PA 18049

5) HOW TO GIVE A NEURO-VASCULAR MASSAGE

Neuro-vascular holding points or receptors, used regularly, are excellent health enhancers. They improve the circulation, especially that of the capillaries, and as you know, anything that improves the circulation improves overall physical and emotional well-being. Impaired circulation, which may be the result of a sedentary life style or poor eating habits or possibly a hereditary predisposition for circulatory disorders, will, over a period of years, greatly reduce the body's ability to function optimally. The body's many organs and systems require a constant supply of nutrients and oxygen in order to repair themselves and to maintain a healthy internal equilibrium.

Improved capillary circulation will also greatly benefit the body's largest organ, the skin. Acne, pallor (extreme or unnatural paleness), dry or oily skin and lifeless hair are but some of the conditions that improve through the regular use of neuro-vascular holding points. Such important body functions as digestion, elimination and respiration also benefit from neuro-vascular massage. Furthermore, improved circulation facilitates the endocrine glands' production of hormones, which regulate the growth, reproduction and nutrient utilization of the body's cells. This, in turn, insures or encourages adequate or optimal cellular activity, normal growth patterns in the formative years and healthy reproductive organs that will permit the continuation and forward the development of a healthy and superior species.

Neuro-vascular holding points are capable of affecting the organs in another important way too.

Our bodies are constantly confronted with toxins, not only those produced within the body, but also those ingested through the digestive tract and inhaled through the respiratory system. Toxins must be continually removed in order for the body to maintain its delicate balance known as homeostasis. An accumulation of toxic wastes within the system impairs bodily functions and can, when excessive, result in death. Improved circulation effects the speedy elimination of backed-up toxic materials and thus allows the body to resume its activities. Lactic acid, a waste that accumulates in the muscles after physical activity, illness or extended periods of inactivity due to a sedentary life style, must also be released. Physical exercise is, of course, the best way to release these toxins. When, however, exercise is not possible or when a supplement to exercise is required, the neuro-vascular holding points are extremely useful and can be included in a full body massage program.

Execution of the neuro-vascular massage is extremely easy, and whether done by yourself or someone else, it is gratifying. If you do the points yourself, there are two possible positions you can assume. One possibility is a reclining position. Lie in bed or on the floor with your knees propped up by pillows or bolster cushions, and support your arms with additional pillows. The second possibility is a crouched position, which is also assumed on a bed or on the floor. Place a folded towel or small compact pillow between your forehead and the floor or bed. Some people find this position easier because the arms are completely relaxed and supported. If you find crouching forward uncomfortable, use the reclining position.

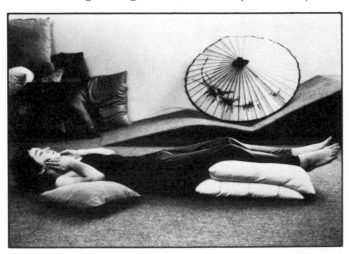

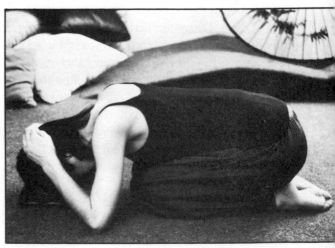

If someone is doing the points for you, refer to the photographs for the most comfortable position. If you are doing the points yourself, be sure your arms are sufficiently propped or supported to prevent the development of muscular fatigue, which will spoil the relaxing and beneficial effects of the neuro-vascular massage.

IMPORTANT CONSIDERATIONS FOR THE NEURO-VASCULAR MASSAGE

- Remove contact lenses.

- Breathe slowly and regularly.

- Make contact with the points by using a light pressure.

- While holding the points, try to keep calm and perfectly still because the slightest movement or turn of the head sends vibrations down your arm which are felt by the receiver.

- Withdraw from the points slowly so as not to jar the receiver.

- If you notice the receiver's eyes batting, it is a sign that the receiver is thinking. Quietly suggest that the receiver try not to think.

- Use the pads of your fingers, not your fingertips.

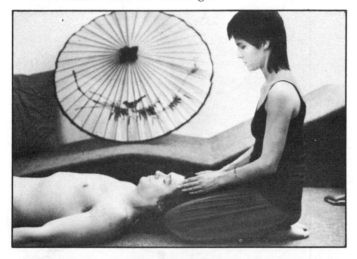

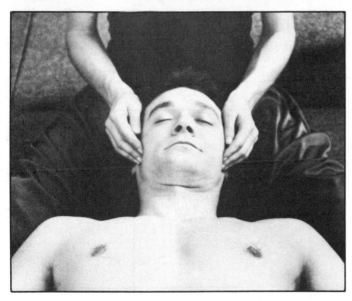

CORRECT

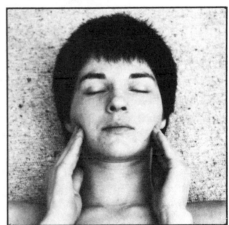

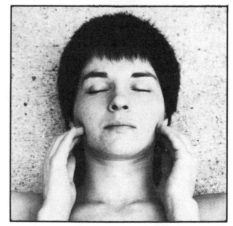

INCORRECT

What to do is extremely simple. Study the following photographs to locate the neuro-vascular holdings points. Feel for a very delicate subcutaneous pulse, i.e. a faint beat under the skin. Hold the pulse for 20-30 seconds and then move on to the next pair of points. Not all the points are found in pairs. Follow the numerical sequence indicated in the photographs. After five or six sessions with the points, you will probably remember their location and sequence so that you will no longer need the book as a guide. The pulses should be held gently and withdrawal must be executed slowly.

Don't be surprised if you fall asleep during this process. You may also notice that you twitch, snore, make nonsensical sounds or release short spurts of words that may or may not make sense. These are all good signs, for they indicate that you are letting go and releasing stored tension.

If someone is doing your points for you, you are more likely to fall asleep because you won't have to concern yourself with maintaining contact with the points. Encourage yourself to relax and let go. Try to free your mind from thought. If you find that impossible, allow thoughts to flow through your mind in a stream of consciousness. Do not focus on any of the thoughts or images, but simply allow them to pass through your mind's eye. Many people have reported achieving a transcendental state of being during neuro-vascular massage. Some people say they feel as if they are floating in and out of consciousness, while others say they have the sensation that they are no longer lying on the mat but floating slightly above it. You may also feel waves of relaxation sweeping over your entire body or through its various parts. If you are really in touch with your body, you may even be able to feel a rush of energy to the organ that corresponds to the points being held. Whatever you feel, it will undoubtedly be a very relaxing and fulfilling experience that you will want to repeat frequently.

The entire process will consume only 10 minutes of your time, and the effects will be well worth your while. You will feel as if you have been off on a long vacation. Your mental alertness will be renewed, your emotional balance restored and your physical well-being refreshed.

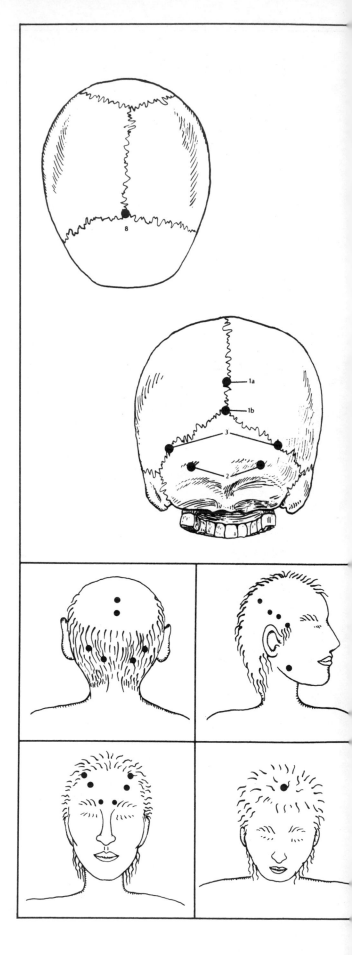

NEURO-VASCULAR HOLDING POINTS

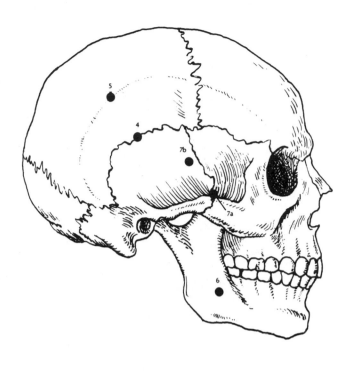

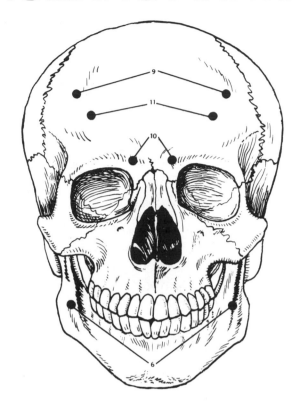

1a Posterior sagittal suture

1b Posterior fontanel

2   Occipital protuberance

3   Lambdoidal suture

4   Squamous suture

5   Parietal eminence

6   Ramus of the jaw

7a Temporal/Sphenoid juncture

7b Squamous portion of temporal bone

8   Anterior fontanel

9   Lateral frontal bone

10 Glabella

11 Frontal eminence

1a Infections, Fevers, Sore throat, Anemia, Tennis elbow

1b Large intestine (diarrhea, constipation, hemmorhoids, etc.), Adrenal Glands (ENERGY STABILIZATION), STRESS CONTROL, Fatigue, Blood sugar problems, Asthma, Allergies, Infection SHOCK from physical or emotional trauma

2   Kidneys, Restlessness, Skin conditions, Low back pain

3   Reproductive/Sexual organ conditions, Hormonal disturbances

4   Spleen, Allergies, Blood sugar problems

5   Small/Large intestine & Digestive disturbances, Kidneys, Reproductive/Sexual organ conditions

6   Stomach, Digestion, Sinus, Eyes, Nose

7a Kidney, Neck

7b Hyper/Hypothyroidism, NERVOUS SYSTEM, Spine

8   Gall Bladder, Liver, Heart & Lung conditons, BRAIN FATIGUE

9   Liver conditions, Headaches

10 Bladder functions & conditions

11 Stomach, Digestion, Bladder conditons, STRESS CONTROL

6) MASSAGE FOR COMMON CHILDHOOD & ADULT COMPLAINTS

Below are some of the various points associated with many everyday complaints. Pain is an alarm system, the body's signal that some function is impaired or threatened. Always consult a holistically oriented physician as soon as you are able, for immediate attention can correct an imbalance before it becomes overwhelming. Use these points to ease any pain or release a blockage until you have the opportunity to consult your doctor, or use them as adjuncts to your doctor's recommendations. These points stimulate the body's natural healing mechanism and thus help to speed up your recovery.

See Neuro-lymphatic Massage Points Chart on page 46, Neuro-vascular Holding Points chart on pages 152 & 153, Meridian Acupuncture Reference Chart on pages 38 & 39 and Foot Reflexology Charts on page 67 & 79 for precise locations of the points utilized in this chapter.

HEADACHE

Each point indicated in the accompanying photographs relates to a particular type of headache. If you are uncertain of the origin of the headache or if the points you have chosen don't seem to be helping, simply do all the points. Trial and error will take care of your headache.

LIVER & GALL BLADDER
Neuro-lymphatic Massage Points

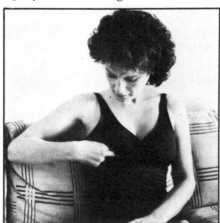

between the 5th & 6th ribs on the right side only

GALL BLADDER
Acupuncture Pressure points

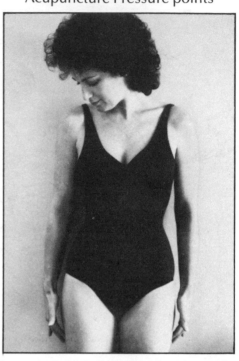

Stand at attention. Gall Bladder 31 is located where the fingertips touch the outside of the thigh.

STOMACH
Neuro-vascular Holding Points

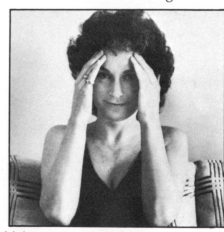

Hold the prominent bulges on your forehead (frontal eminence).

EYESTRAIN

Use your thumbs for the upper orbit and your fingers for the lower orbit of each eye. Apply pressure and hold for 3-5 seconds. Lymphatic massage points are located on the inside edge of the humerus bone. Use your thumb for these points.

UPPER ORBIT PRESSURE POINTS

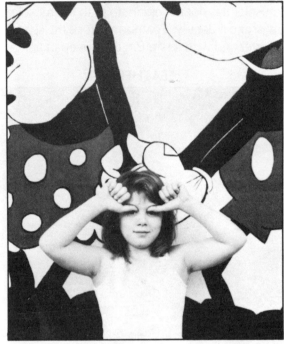

Apply firm pressure

KIDNEY
Neuro-lymphatic Massage Points

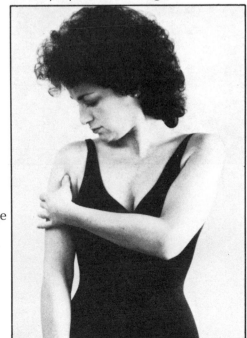

Massage both arms.

INDIGESTION

Indigestion can result from the malfunctioning of one or more of several digestive organs. Note the photographs for the exact location of each of the points. Apply pressure or massage the appropriate area(s) until you experience relief. Sometimes a period of as much as two to five minutes is necessary to relieve the discomfort. These points may also be stimulated prior to and during a meal in order to assist the deficient organ(s) and possibly to avoid indigestion.

STOMACH
Neuro-lymphatic Massage Points

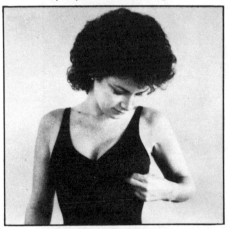

between the 5th & 6th ribs on the left side only

LIVER & GALL BLADDER
Neuro-lymphatic Massage Points

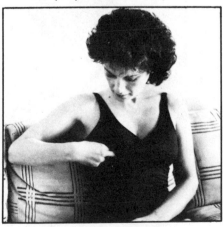

between the 5th & 6th ribs on the right side only

155

LOW BACK PAIN

The neuro-lymphatics for the lower back are located on the inside of the thigh. Use your elbow or your fingers to massage thoroughly and with a firm pressure the entire area depicted in the accompanying photograph. Usually one to three minutes are required to bring relief, although sometimes relief comes in thirty seconds.

SMALL INTESTINE
Neuro-lymphatic Massage Points

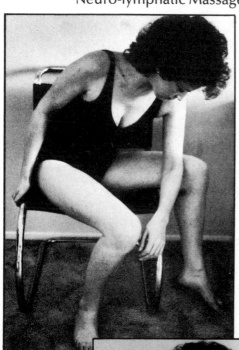

Massage firmly the lower half of the inside of the thigh.

CALF CRAMPS

When you experience cramps or spasms in your calf muscle, you want to relax or sedate the mechanisms within the belly of the muscle. Feathering from the belly of the muscle toward the origin and insertion will sedate the muscle sufficiently to stop the spasm. Feathering is a very light technique. Try to evoke the same sensations a feather would if it were drawn over your calf muscle. It is not necessary to grab the muscle or to massage it deeply. Feathering stops the spasm sooner and with less effort than deep massage.

FEATHERING

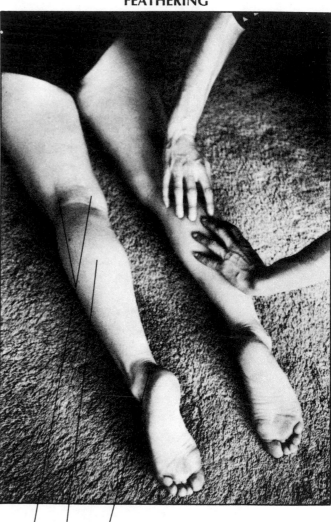

Origin   Belly   Insertion

TENNIS ELBOW

This common tennis injury is sometimes more complicated than you would expect. If the neuro-vascular holding points and the neuro-lymphatic massage points shown in the following photographs do not correct the conditions, you may well have a sacral fixation. Try bringing your knees up to your chest and rolling from side to side on the floor. If, after a reasonable time, no results are achieved, see a chiropractor.

SPLEEN
Neuro-lymphatic Massage Point

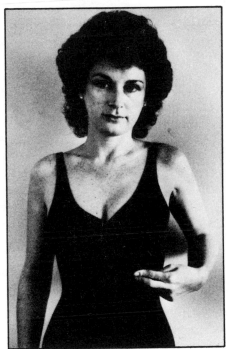

between the 7th & 8th ribs on the left side only

SPLEEN
Neuro-vascular Holding Point

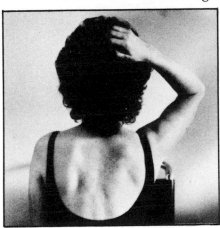

Locate this point 1½ inches above the posterior fontanel.

LOW ENERGY

Massage the two sets of points indicated in the photographs. One-and-a-half minutes for each set of points will usually be sufficient to clear a foggy mind and to supply you with more energy. These points are useful for long-distance driving, for studying, for sleepy attacks at concerts or for any occasion that would normally drive you to coffee. The points in the first set are located two-and-a-half inches above and one inch on either side of the navel. Massage deep into the abdomen, just below the rib cage. These points stimulate the functioning of your adrenal glands. Do not massage the adrenal points too close to bedtime because you may find yourself unable to sleep. The points of the second set are located on either side of the chest from the clavicle to the arm pit. Massage these neuro-lymphatics firmly, even though they may feel tender or a bit painful. The sensitivity will decrease as your alertness increases. These points correspond to the brain.

TRIPLE WARMER
Neuro-lymphatic Massage Points

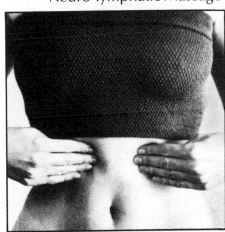

Locate these points under the rib cage.

CENTRAL
Neuro-lymphatic Massage Points

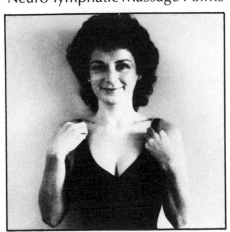

SORE THROAT

Below you will find three different approaches for deterring the progress or speeding the recovery of a sore throat. The neuro-lymphatic massage point for the throat is located on the left side of the chest between the seventh and eighth ribs. The point will be tender when you massage it, so you will know when you are in the correct location. The neuro-vascular holding point for a sore throat is located one-half inches above the Posterior fontanel, which was the baby soft spot on the back of the head. See Illustrations on pages 152 & 153 for the location of this point. Use the pads of your fingers to locate the point on your head. Be sure you feel a pulse under the scalp, and then hold this point for 1-3 minutes at a time as needed. The foot reflex point for a sore throat is located at the base of the big toe on the bottom of each foot. This point will also be tender to a firm touch. Be brave. Massage the base of the big toe with a very firm pressure. Try to endure the discomfort because the pain you may feel from the toe is going to be of a much shorter duration than that from the sore throat. These reflex points are particularly effective if used at the first sign of a sore throat. Use the points frequently, every fifteen minutes if necessary, and you may not even get a sore throat. If you begin to implement the points after the sore throat has settled in, you can achieve a speedier recovery, but usually cannot make it disappear.

Neuro-vascular Holding Point

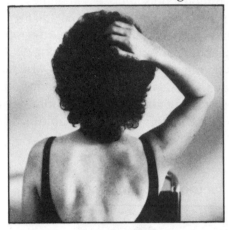

Located 1½ inches above the Posterior fontanel

FOOT REFLEXOLOGY

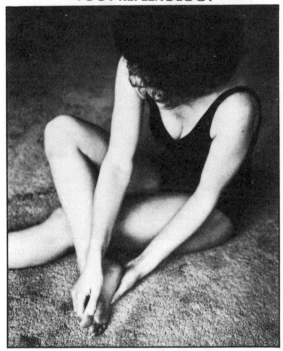

Massage firmly.

SPLEEN
Neuro-lymphatic Massage Point

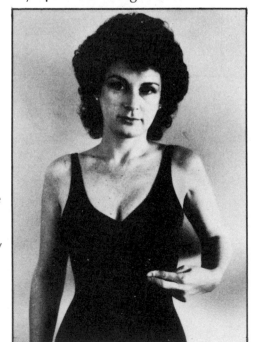

between the 7th & 8th ribs on the left side only

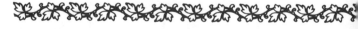

TOOTHACHE

Firmly massage and apply pressure to the inside edge of the humerus bone. If your toothache is on the right side of your mouth, massage your right arm; if it's on the left side, massage your left arm. You will undoubtedly find an extremely painful spot on the inside edge of your arm bone. That's the point. Work it hard. It will hurt, but the pain in your tooth will usually disappear in one or two minutes. The photograph shows a dark band of points. Try all of them. Usually one or two of these points will be more painful than the rest. These are the points on which to concentrate your pressure and massage. Be sure to consult your dentist. Remember, pain is the body's alarm system letting you know something is not right.

KIDNEY
Neuro-lymphatic Massage Points

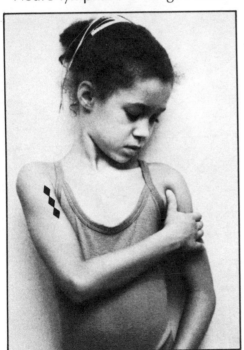

Massage firmly.

SMOKER'S LUNG

Massage the lymphatic points on either side of the sternum between the third and fourth as well as the fourth and fifth ribs, and/or apply firm pressure to each of the points indicated on the forearm for 7-10 seconds. Heavy smokers of cigarettes or marijuana should do these points four to six times a day.

LUNG
Neuro-lymphatic Massage Points

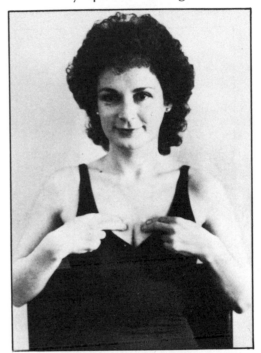

Massage near the sternum.

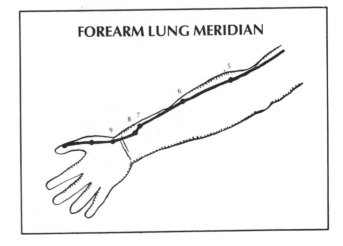

FOREARM LUNG MERIDIAN

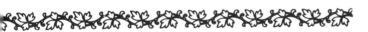

DRINKER'S LIVER

Massage the intercostal space between the fifth and sixth ribs on the right side of the chest only. Use firm pressure and massage for 2-3 minutes four to six times a day. You may also hold the neuro-vascular point on the top of your head for 1-3 minutes four to six times a day. This technique helps to increase the flow of blood, nutrients and energy to your liver.

LIVER
Neuro-lymphatic Massage Points

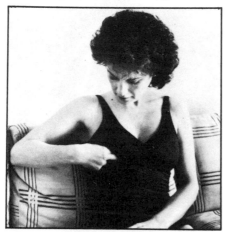

between the 5th & 6th ribs on the right side only

LIVER
Neuro-vascular Holding Point

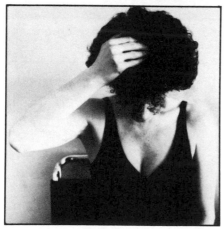

Locate this point on the Anterior fontanel
(baby's soft spot on top of the head)

CONSTIPATION/DIARRHEA

Thoroughly massage, with a firm pressure, the area indicated on the side of the thigh. Massage up to eliminate constipation and down to eliminate diarrhea. Massage when attempting to move your bowels, as well as once in the morning and once in the evening before going to sleep. Of course, plenty of bran, exercise and water are also factors important to proper functioning of the bowels.

LARGE INTESTINE
Neuro-lymphatic Massage Points

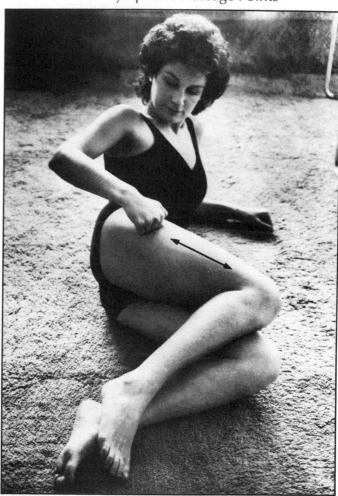

Massage both legs

SLEEPLESSNESS

Hold the neuro-vascular holding points located on the forehead. Feel for the pulse and hold the points for five minutes or longer. Usually within a few minutes you will begin to feel relaxed enough to fall asleep. You can also sedate your adrenal glands by holding the neuro-vascular holding point on the posterior fontanel. See page 153 for more information.

STOMACH
Neuro-vascular Holding Points

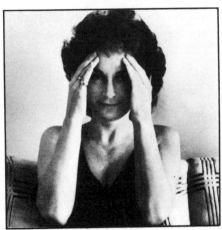

The frontal eminence points affect the emotional center of the brain

TRIPLE WARMER
Neuro-vascular Holding Point

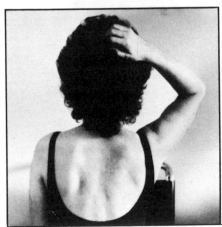

Locate this point on the posterior fontanel

SINUS CONDITIONS

Firmly massage the upper inner edge of the arm's humerus bone. Pressure applied to the orbits of the eyes also benefits sinus conditions. Firm pressure to the maxilla bones on either side of the nose is also very beneficial. Helpful too, are Large Intestine 20, and Lung 11. Hold each application of pressure for 7-10 seconds.

KIDNEY
Neuro-lymphatic Massage Points

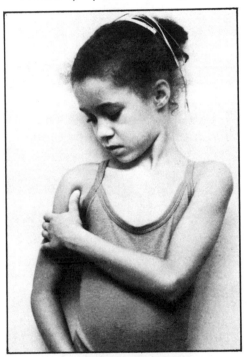

Massage both arms

LOWER ORBIT PRESSURE POINTS

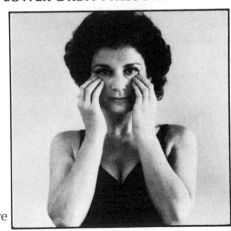

Apply firm pressure

LARGE INTESTINE
Acupuncture Pressure Points

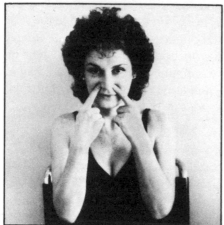

Apply firm pressure to Large intestine 20

LARGE INTESTINE & LUNG
Acupuncture Pressure Points

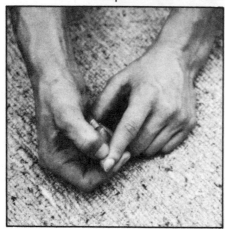

Apply firm
pressure to
Large intestine 1

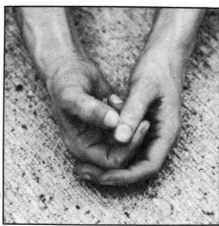

Apply firm
pressure to
Lung 11

SHOULDER & NECK TENSION

The following acupuncture points can be used with very firm thumb pressure for 7-10 seconds and repeated three times: Gall Bladder 20, Gall Bladder 21, Large Intestine 16 and Small Intestine 11. Of course, massaging the origin, belly and insertion of the upper trapezius muscle will also contribute to the release of shoulder and neck tension.

GALL BLADDER
Acupuncture Pressure Points

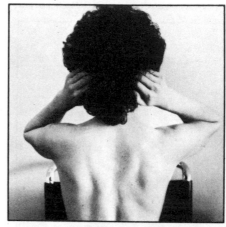

Apply firm pressure to Gall Bladder 20

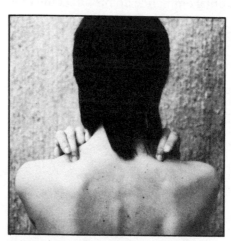

Apply firm pressure to Gall Bladder 21

LARGE INTESTINE
Acupuncture Pressure Points

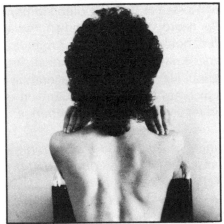

Apply firm pressure to Large intestine 16

SMALL INTESTINE
Acupuncture Pressure Points

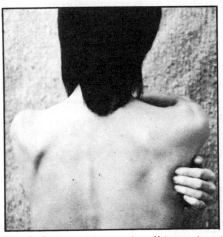

Apply firm pressure to Small intestine 11

EMOTIONALLY UPSETTING SITUATIONS

Hold the frontal eminences on the forehead for up to ten minutes. Often two or three minutes are sufficient. The posterior fontanel, (the baby's soft spot on the back of the head), corresponds to the adrenal glands, which are always in need of normalization after a traumatic event. Hold this point for 2-10 minutes, depending upon the severity of the situation. You will know when you have held both the frontal eminence points and the adrenal points a sufficient length of time, for you will suddenly realize that the problem which was so upsetting no longer seems to be disturbing your psyche. Feel for a light pulse in the correct location.

STOMACH
Neuro-vascular Holding Points

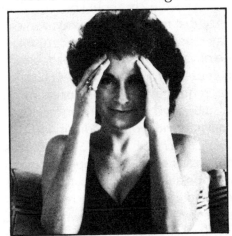

Hold the prominent bulges on your forehead
(frontal eminence)

TRIPLE WARMER
Neuro-vascular Holding Point

Locate this point on the Posterior fontanel

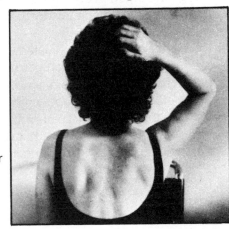

7) PRIVATE MOMENTS IN PUBLIC PLACES

Most people cope continually with some sort of nagging physical problem, be it headaches, constipation or digestive disturbances, or with a more serious matter like glaucoma, ulcers or liver or kidney malfunctioning. There are pressure points and techniques that, when implemented on a daily basis, will help to right or stabilize most conditions of ill health. Employing the correct pressure points for your condition will encourage your body's natural healing mechanism to work more effectively and quickly, and thereby speed up your recovery or stabilize your condition. Most conditions respond if you are diligent and work your points four to six times a day. This may seem like a lot of work, but it's not. When you consider how much time you spend daily taking pills or worrying needlessly about your condition, you will realize that ten to fifteen minutes spread out over a day is very little time indeed. Aim to make the use of your points a matter of habit. Schedule their use as you see fit for your lifestyle, but make it as requisite as breathing or eating. The points can also be used whenever you feel discomfort associated with your condition.

HOW TO USE THESE POINTS: Hold, massage or apply pressure to the appropriate points for your condition at least four to six times a day. If you utilize the points less than the recommended frequency, you will get slower results, although you will still experience some assistance and relief. The secret is to work the points for your condition many times daily for 1-3 minutes at a time. Frequent applications keep a constant flow of energy, blood, nutrients and lymph circulating to or through the organ in question so that the body's natural healing mechanism can function more efficiently.

If you have a condition associated with any of these pressure or massage points, you will probably find that the appropriate point will be tender or a little painful. Massage or apply pressure to the point even though it hurts. You will not harm the tissue or muscle at its location, but you will help its associated organ. You will notice as you massage or apply pressure to the point that the tenderness will lessen as your condition improves.

Whenever neuro-vascular holding points are recommended, hold the points for 1-3 minutes, four to six times a day. The neuro-lymphatic massage points should be massaged 30 seconds at a time four to six times a day. Acupuncture pressure points should receive pressure for a period of one minute.

For clarification of the following points see the Neuro-vascular Holding Points Chart on pages 152 & 153, the Neuro-lymphatic Massage Points Chart on page 46 and the Meridian Acupuncture Reference Chart on pages 38 & 39.

EYES & EARS & NOSE & TEETH

Any condition related to these organs will improve from frequent massaging of the inner edge of the humerus bone in the upper arm. Massage, very firmly, the area indicated in the photograph.

KIDNEY
Neuro-lymphatic Massage Points

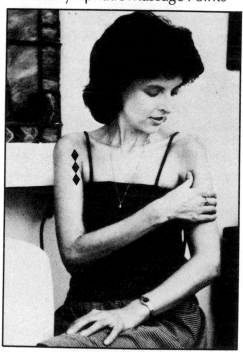

Massage firmly into the bone

GALL BLADDER CONDITIONS

Insert your middle finger into the intercostal space between the fifth and sixth ribs, which are located below the right breast or pectoralis muscle. Firmly massage the area indicated in the photograph.

GALL BLADDER
Neuro-lymphatic Massage Points

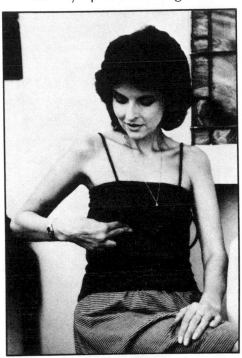

Massage firmly

REPRODUCTIVE ORGAN CONDITIONS

Apply firm thumbnail pressure or firm thumb pressure to the base of the middle fingernail at the terminal acupuncture point, and apply thumb pressure into the point at the center of the crease of the elbow. Never apply great pressure at a joint, only one that feels good and comfortable.

CIRCULATION/SEX
Acupuncture Pressure Points

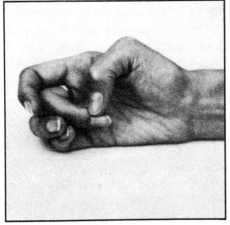

Circulation/Sex 9

CIRCULATION/SEX
Acupuncture Pressure Points

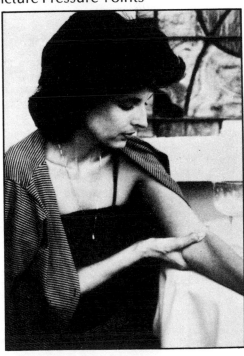

Circulation/Sex 3

ADRENAL IMBALANCE

The neuro-vascular holding point for the adrenal glands is located on the back of the head where the baby's soft spot was located. These points will help to normalize adrenal gland conditions. The lymphatic massage points for the adrenal glands are located one inch to the side of and two-and-a-half inches up from the navel. Use your middle finger, braced by the fingers on either side of it, to massage deeply into these points. It is easier to massage one side at a time when in public. These massage points should not be done before going to bed, for stimulation of the adrenal glands will keep you awake and alert. These points are useful for studying, keeping awake at concerts, driving long distances and getting a quick pick-me-up at the office.

TRIPLE WARMER
Neuro-vascular Holding Point

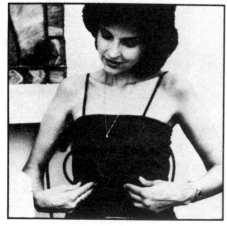

Hold lightly & feel for a pulse

Neuro-lymphatic Massage Points

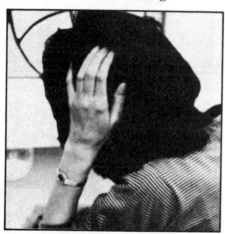

Massage firmly

BLADDER CONDITIONS

Bladder conditions caused by nervousness are greatly benefited by the frontal eminence neuro-vascular holding points. Other bladder conditions respond well to the bladder points located between the eyes, as well as the above mentioned points.

STOMACH
Neuro-vascular Holding Points

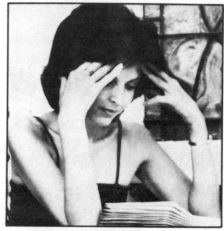

Hold lightly & feel for a pulse

BLADDER
Neuro-vascular Holding Points

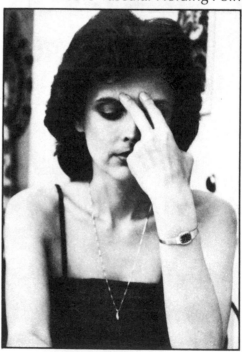

Hold lightly & feel for a pulse

SMALL INTESTINE CONDITIONS

The lymphatic massage points on the inside of the lower thigh are quite helpful for conditions of the intestinal tract and for low back pain. Use your fingers or your elbow to firmly massage the appropriate area of the thigh.

SMALL INTESTINE
Neuro-lymphatic Massage Points

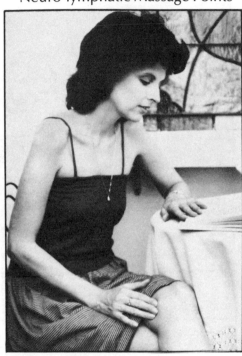

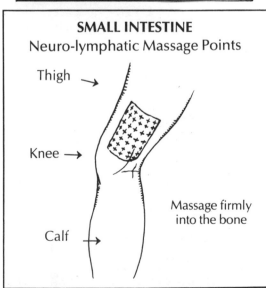

SMALL INTESTINE
Neuro-lymphatic Massage Points

Thigh →

Knee →

Massage firmly
into the bone

Calf →

STOMACH CONDITIONS

The frontal eminence neuro-vascular holding points are excellent for stomach disorders, particularly those of the nervous type. The stomach acupuncture pressure points #36 on the leg below the knee are also useful. The latter points can be done more easily in public than the frontal eminence points, although they can be done quite easily while reading at your desk.

STOMACH
Neuro-vascular Holding Points

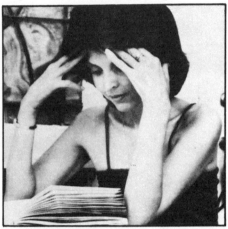

Hold lightly & feel for a pulse

STOMACH
Acupuncture Pressure Points

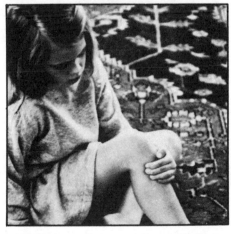

Apply firm pressure to Stomach 36

THYROID FUNCTION

Place the three middle fingers of one hand on the neuro-vascular holding points for the thyroid. The points can be held quite casually whether you are in a seated or standing position. The thyroid gland regulates the body's metabolic rate. Metabolic processes must function at the proper rate in order for all other systems to function effectively and efficiently. Hold these points gently enough to feel a light pulse with your finger tips. Do not apply pressure, for these are holding points, _not_ pressure points.

TRIPLE WARMER
Neuro-vascular Holding Points

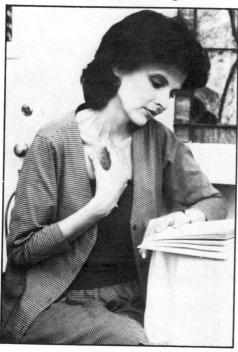

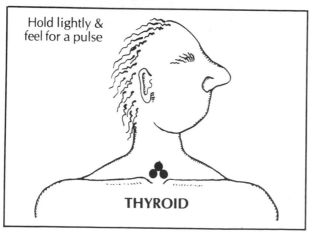

Hold lightly &
feel for a pulse

THYROID

PANCREAS CONDITIONS

The neuro-vascular holding points for the pancreas are particularly beneficial to people with sugar metabolism problems. Liver points should also be done in conjunction with the pancreas points.

SPLEEN
Neuro-vascular Holding Points

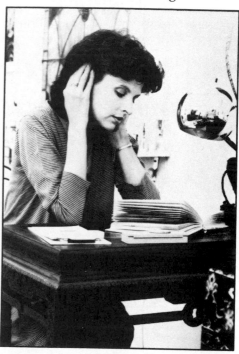

Hold Pancreas points lightly & feel for a pulse

LIVER
Neuro-vascular Holding Points

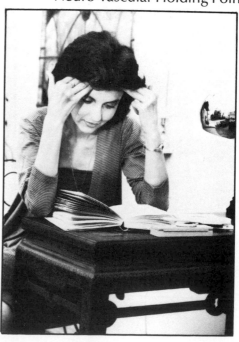

Hold lightly
& feel for
a pulse
at the hair
line

LUNG CONDITIONS

Use your thumbnail to apply firm pressure into the terminal acupuncture points for the Lung Meridian. Application of a very firm pressure also benefits these points. Do both thumbnails, unless you know specifically which lung is involved. Firm pressure into the pad of your thumb is also a good method of improving the flow of energy to the lungs.

LUNG
Acupuncture Pressure Points

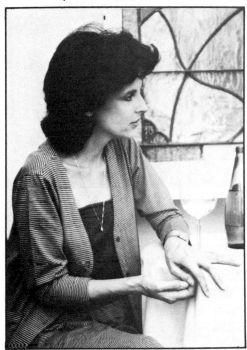

Apply firm pressure to Lung 11

LUNG
Acupuncture Pressure Points

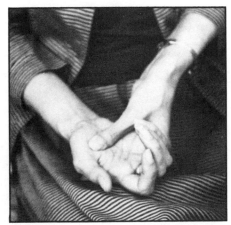

Apply firm pressure to Lung 10

LIVER POINTS

Spleen 6 on the lower inside edge of the shinbones is useful for liver disturbances. These points can also be done very inconspicuously in public. Apply firm pressure.

SPLEEN
Acupuncture Pressure Points

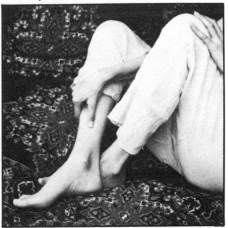

Apply firm pressure to Spleen 6

KIDNEY POINTS

Spleen 6 is beneficial to the kidneys too. Kidney 27 is another useful and easily accessible point. Use these points regularly to assist the kidneys. Don't forget to drink plenty of water. Apply firm pressure to Spleen 6 and massage Kidney 27.

KIDNEY
Neuro-lymphatic Massage Points

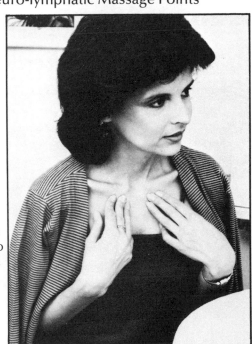

Massage firmly into the bone

HEART & CIRCULATORY CONDITIONS

Using a firm pressure, squeeze and twist the base of the fingernail for the terminal acupuncture points of the Heart and Circulation/Sex Meridians. Use your thumbnail to apply firm pressure to the points at the bases of the nails. You will know when you are on the point because it will be quite tender. Tolerate a little discomfort for a few minutes a day to avoid perhaps years of discomfort. This is a primitive form of acupuncture. It is quite effective.

HEART
Acupuncture Pressure Points

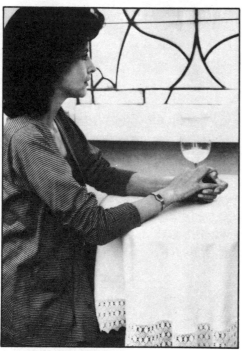

Apply firm pressure to Heart 9

CIRCULATION/SEX
Acupuncture Pressure Points

Apply firm pressure to Circulation/Sex 9

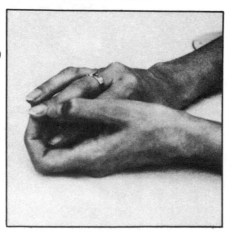

SPLEEN POINT FOR INFECTIONS

The neuro-vascular holding point for the spleen is useful for colds, flu or any infection you may contract. This point assists the immune system in its battle. Contact the holding point one-half inches above the baby soft spot on the back of the head.

SPLEEN
Neuro-vascular Holding Points

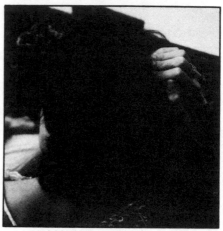

Hold lightly & feel for a pulse

CONSTIPATION

Apply firm penetrating pressure into the metacarpal bone of the index finger at the point just below the "V" where the thumb metacarpal meets the index metacarpal. This point should also be utilized while attempting to move your bowels. It is helpful to place your feet on a foot rest that is approximately three inches lower than the toilet seat. This is the correct position for efficient bowel movements. Toilet seats may be comfortable to sit on, but they are impractical because it is natural to assume a squatting position when moving the bowels.

LARGE INTESTINE
Acupuncture Pressure Points

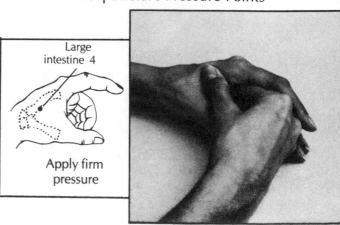

Large intestine 4

Apply firm pressure

CHAPTER VI

Factors That Increase The Benefits of Massage

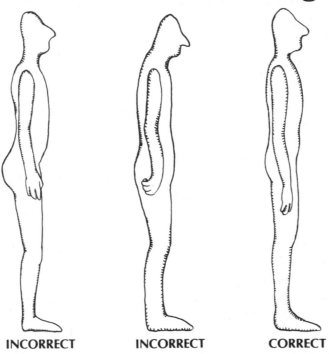

| INCORRECT | INCORRECT | CORRECT |

INTRODUCTION

In order to benefit fully and thoroughly from regular sessions of massage, you must integrate its magic into a complete program for good health. The seven sections in this chapter will introduce you to some of the necessary complements to massage therapy.

Granted, massage alone is capable of significantly upgrading your emotional and physical health and of improving or curing both chronic and acute conditions; but only a synthesis of proper diet, nutritional supplements, correct posture, regular exercise, meditation, homoeopathic medicine, general health aides and massage can achieve your long-term goal of good health. I hope the information in this chapter will stimulate your interest and set you in the right direction in your search for good health through eclectic massage.

1)POSTURE

Your posture reflects how you feel about yourself and how you see yourself in relation to other people. If you have a positive, self-confident approach to life, your posture is likely to be erect. A slumped posture, on the other hand, usually indicates a defeatist, negative attitude. The way you relate to yourself and others also determines how much your posture will succumb to the earth's constant pull of gravity. Gravity is both your enemy and your friend. Without gravity life on this planet would be impossible, but gravity also subjects you to a constant downward pull that can easily overcome you and produce an extremely exaggerated, slumped posture. As if that isn't enough, you also have to cope with postural deviations caused by other events beyond your control, like accidents, deaths, pollution, noise and all the annoyances of a modern, indifferent, technological society. It is, therefore, easy to understand why optimum posture is not so easily achieved. If you also consider that you were not taught how to walk, sit down, get up, reach or bend over, it is absolutely amazing that you're doing as well as you are. Imagine what a little correctional training could do for you!

In light of the overwhelming odds against good posture, the logical question to ask is what you can do to correct your understandable deficiencies. There is a method known as the Alexander Technique that offers a working solution to the problem. The Alexander Technique evolved over a period of ten years through concentrated effort by its originator, F. Matthias Alexander. Since the late nineteenth century, people from all walks of life have been benefiting from his discoveries. Among the more renowned people who have praised him and used his methods are Sir Charles Sherrington, John Dewey, Lilly Langtry, Professor Nikolaas Tinbergen, Aldous Huxley, Gertrude Stein's brother Leo, and George Bernard Shaw. The Alexander Technique is very popular among dancers, singers, actors and musicians, because proper posture is of utmost importance when you want to be the best in your field. For this reason, too, scientists, doctors and concerned lay people have employed the Alexander Technique. Why shouldn't each of us strive to be the best we can be?

Correct posture is basic to optimum health. If your neck is thrust forward and down, if your chest sags and your back is humped at the shoulders and arched in the lower lumbar region, how can the necessary blood, energy and nutrients reach your internal organs or muscles? Such a deformed posture weighs heavily on your internal organs, especially on your lungs, and hinders the functioning of the digestive and circulatory systems. Many conditions, including headaches, eye problems, hearing loss, digestive disturbances, chronic shoulder and neck tension, lower back pain and mental fatigue are all closely related to poor posture. Many other ailments also respond to improved posture. Contact a teacher trained in the Alexander Technique and begin lessons. You will be surprised at the number of your physical and emotional complaints that will disappear or lessen after a few lessons. Allow an Alexander teacher to reeducate you by correcting your postural habits and movements. Instructors will begin by creating an awareness of the bad habits you are now practicing and will then teach you how to correct and replace them with new postural habits and movements.

If you are interested in improving your physical and emotional lot, I very emphatically recommend that you now begin to take Alexander lessons in order to correct your postural deviations. Massage can and does improve the posture, as well as the flow of blood, nutrients and energy to internal organs and muscles. The improvement, however, is often temporary, because most people have not been sufficiently reeducated as to their abnormal holding and movement patterns. Ideally, massage therapy should come after or in conjunction with your reeducation in correct postural alignment. Don't misinterpret. Massage is always helpful, but it will have a more lasting and profound effect on your entire system if your posture is optimal.

Attempting to improve your health without correcting faulty posture is like trying to build a house on a lop-sided foundation and around a poorly constructed frame. Such a house would not do well under stress and strain. How can you, therefore, expect your body to react favorably to tension and disease with poor posture and alignment as your foundation and frame?

2)EXERCISE

Strenuous exercise is a marvelous way to lose weight, firm flabby tissue, build muscles, improve circulation, clear the lymphatic system and generally improve your health. Unfortunately, many of us are so out of shape that starting a rigorous exercise program is often disastrous. Too many people end up with more aches and pains than they had prior to their enthusiastic embarkment on a new exercise program. It's no wonder, for attempting a serious exercise program with poor alignment can only lead to injury. If your shoulders are rounded, your upper back hunched over and your lower back arched, you are no longer using the muscles of your body as you should. A body this much out of alignment cannot tolerate the demands that strenuous exercise puts on the skeletal and muscular systems. Attempting to do too much too soon and choosing the wrong kind of exercise for your body type are two other common reasons why exercise often proves to be detrimental rather than beneficial. So, before you embark on an exercise program, treat yourself first to a series of Alexander lessons. Then choose the proper form of exercise for your body type and lifestyle.

If you feel that your posture is quite good, as I did, you will be surprised how much more Alexander lessons can teach you about the many subtle adjustments and significant changes necessary for your body to achieve optimum posture and health. During and after your lessons you will experience a new-found freedom of movement and grace, as well as a significant improvement in your emotional equilibrium.

Before I suggest some preferred types of exercises, allow me to say a few words about jogging, our nation's favorite way to exercise. Jogging can work wonderfully to tone your body, strengthen your muscles and improve your vascular system. It can also do a lot of harm. Most people out there jogging are not fit for it. Unless your body is lithe and your posture close to perfect, you should forget about running your body to health. People with large bones, stalky builds, poor posture, excess weight or large breasts should not be jogging. Every step you take jars your entire spinal column and all the joints in your legs. In addition, your internal organs also take quite a beating on each successive impact. The medical profession is making millions of dollars annually on self-inflicted injuries related to jogging, not to mention injuries resulting from accidents with moving vehicles. Jogging on concrete is absolutely out of the question for the above-mentioned reasons. Jogging in or near traffic and inhaling those carbon-monoxide fumes is totally ridiculous. Unless you can run on a wooden track or on turf in a park or in the country, forget it. You'd probably be better off not running at all.

An excellent substitute for jogging is rebounding on a small trampoline. Set up your trampoline near an open window or outdoors. Then jog, kick, twist and jump to your heart's content, without experiencing any of the negative side-effects of jogging. Rebounding is easy to do, and it exercises every muscle and strengthens every cell in your body. Most important, trampolining is fun, and all you need is ten minutes twice a day to make it profitable exercise. Any more than ten minutes at a time does not significantly increase the benefits. Rebound first thing in the morning to get your adrenal glands and circulation going for the whole day. Rebound before meals to curb your appetite. Rebound while watching television. Rebound if you're feeling tired. Rebound any time at all. In a matter of three days you will be hooked and loving it. Rebounding is safe. It's economical, as a trampoline is a one-time investment. It's not time-consuming, and it strengthens and tones your entire body. Besides all that, it's lots of FUN.

There are many different ways to exercise, but I am only going to recommend exercises that develop both sides of your body equally. That leaves out tennis, handball, racketball, baseball and the like, because such sports demand the use of one side of the body more than the other. They thus encourage unnatural tension and strain on the skeletal and muscular systems. Instead, consider exercises like jogging on turf or wooden track, very fast walking with arms swinging freely, trampolining, yoga, Tai Chi Chuan, roller-skating, swimming, body-building or cross-country skiing.

Yoga and Tai Chi Chuan are excellent for toning and stretching muscles, for improving balance and for effecting relaxation, but neither do as much for the vascular system as more active forms of exercise. Therefore, if you practice yoga or Tai Chi Chuan daily, you would do well also to trampoline or practice any of the other suggested types of exercise.

Exercise is necessary, though usually difficult for most of us to do regularly. If you haven't found a form of exercise that comes to you easily, consider trampolining. Whatever you choose, before you pursue it, remember to get your postural problems corrected, if possible, with an Alexander teacher. The cost is well worth the savings in long-term medical bills that will be avoided.

Massage, a passive form of exercise, affects our system in much the same way as active, willful forms of exercise. The effects are not as profound, but circulation, lymph flow and muscle tone do improve. Massage can even exercise and free tension from the joints of the body through the use of mechanotherapy techniques. Mechanotherapy can be passive, in which case the therapist does the joint manipulation; active, in which case the receiver willfully puts the joints through the range of motion; or resisted, in which case the massage therapist or the receiver resists the movements. Unless a person is extremely ill or disabled, massage cannot serve as a substitute for exercise. It can, however, complement and enhance the beneficial effects of an exercise program. Because regular exercise lowers tension levels and generally improves body functions, the massage therapist can reach deep-seated tensions rather than superficial ones.

---

3)FOODS FOR OPTIMUM HEALTH

I am concerned about your health. I want you to feel better, look better, and achieve *your* level of optimum health. The purpose of this section is to teach you which foods produce optimum health. I am also concerned about world hunger, pollution, and animal abuse. It is a wonderful twist of fate that the very things I am going to teach you about food will also enable you to contribute in a very personal way toward the healing of our planet. This section was written as "food for thought" primarily for people who know little about how foods fight world hunger, pollution, and animal abuse and disease. You, too, may be concerned about these issues but may feel helpless to address them. But you aren't helpless. You *can* participate, on an individual, grass roots basis, by simply choosing to eat only certain foods. You won't have

to attend meetings, make donations, or join demonstrations. The beauty of it is that while you are healing the world, you'll be healing yourself.

What to eat and/or what not to eat has become one of the most controversial subjects of the past few decades. The science of nutrition is, at best, confusing because individual nutritional requirements vary so greatly. Age, lifestyle, stress levels, geographic location, genetic weaknesses, sex, and diet are only some of the influencing factors. Authority figures (parents, doctors, scientists, and the government) are either uneducated, personally biased, or too entangled with big industry to be of any assistance. Studies evaluating and comparing the health and diet of various societies (including Western vegetarian Seventh-Day Adventists) indicate that a vegetarian society (one that consumes no meat, fowl, or fish) enjoys significantly better health than those societies that consume excessive amounts of meat, fowl, and fish. Research also indicates that as consumption of animal foods increases, disease, premature aging, and premature death increase proportionately. What this means is, the closer your diet is to total vegetarianism (no flesh, dairy or eggs), the healthier you will be. Let's not forget, a diet closer to vegetarianism will not only lead to optimum health for you, it will also help alleviate world hunger, pollution, and animal abuse. These issues will be dealt with more fully later on in this section.

Human beings, considered by some experts to be omnivores, have long digestive tracts that are typical of vegetarian species. A long digestive tract facilitates the digestion of high-fiber plant foods because they require more transit time in the small intestine for maximum nutrient assimilation. Species that consume primarily animal protein (carnivores) have short digestive tracts to facilitate the speedy exit of the fiberless, concentrated protein foods they eat. Human beings have a twenty-five- to thirty-foot digestive tract, amply supplied with carbohydrate-digesting enzymes.

Our extensive digestive tracts are not well suited to the consumption of flesh or other animal foods. Fiberless foods such as flesh, other animal products (dairy and eggs), and refined foods remain too long in our digestive tract, resulting in fermentation and putrefaction which is toxic to our entire system. This toxicity is not enough to kill us immediately, but it does lower our vitality and contributes to the development of disease. Animal food products, because they are high in fats and cholesterol, also encourage the development of diabetes, heart disease, and cancer, diseases that plague modern nations known for their high consumption of animal protein and refined foods. Our teeth are best suited for grinding. Our hands are gathering hands; they are not clawed for ripping flesh. The anatomical and biological evidence speaks for itself. We are designed to be vegetarians even though we can eat like omnivores and survive. Obviously, eating animal foods three times a day, as people usually do in this culture, is not the best choice for optimum health.

Why hasn't this information been widely publicized? The answer, unfortunately, is in large part monetary. So much money has been invested in the animal and agricultural food industries that neither the industries nor the government will encourage massive, radical dietary changes. Vegetarianism, or a diet as close to it as possible, would be beneficial to our health, our planet, and all life on it, but our entire economic structure would be devastated. History proves that radical but necessary changes always occur painfully and slowly. Economic stability is fine, but not if it contributes to world hunger, pollution, animal suffering, and less than optimum health. The animal food industries and those industries producing refined foods can only be significantly reduced or eliminated by the combined efforts of caring people.

The correlation between disease and diet is becoming more and more evident. Many people are voluntarily consuming less animal protein. Some have abandoned the consumption of flesh foods. Health-food stores and restaurants selling unprocessed, unrefined whole foods are flourishing. National health organizations are openly discouraging the consumption of animal protein and refined foods. Many doctors are becoming less traditional, suggesting a diet of whole foods and a drastic reduction in the consumption of animal foods. Some doctors recommend the total elimination of animal foods. The shift toward a vegetarian society has already begun. More than ten years in the field of holistic health has led me repeatedly to the same inevitable conclusion: Optimum health can be obtained by becoming a whole-foods vegetarian or as close to a whole-foods vegetarian as possible.

If you are not willing or able to become a total vegetarian, you can consume animal foods as infrequently as possible. Start by consuming each category of animal food no more than once a week. Your body will make it perfectly clear to you that you were getting sick and old before your time by consuming animal foods and refined foods three times a day. When you feel comfortable with these changes, consider reducing your consumption of animal foods and refined foods to a maximum of twice a week. Who knows, you may feel so happy with your newfound health and youthfulness that you will decide to become a whole-foods vegetarian. Even if you don't, you will discover that maintaining a diet as close to vegetarianism as possible is an excellent way to achieve improved health.

Make your choice now. Do you want to be 70 percent healthier, 80 percent healthier, 90 percent healthier? To be or not to be a vegetarian is *not* the question! The question is, how close to being a vegetarian you are willing or able to come. (Don't get me wrong; if you want to become a total vegetarian, please do.) Everyone wants and needs to do as much as possible for their health. All you have to do is eat less animal foods and eat more whole foods. The choice is *yours*. It is important to note that in conjunction with the significant reduction or elimination of animal foods, it is equally imperative to reduce or eliminate the consumption of refined foods. (Don't panic, there are plenty of delicious desserts that can be purchased or made from delicious whole foods.) Whole, unprocessed, vegetarian foods can best help you achieve optimum health.

HOW AND WHY HUMAN BEINGS BEGAN EATING FLESH AND ANIMAL PRODUCTS

Human life undoubtedly evolved in a tropical climate where the heat and lush vegetation provided the necessities for human survival. Fruits, vegetables, seeds, nuts, and grains grew plentifully. Nomadic tribes probably lived on only these foods. Eventually these tribes settled and became agricultural, thus ensuring a more constant food supply. Gathering wild foods supplemented their agricultural efforts and provided variety. Plant foods provided the fiber, protein, enzymes, and other nutrients best suited for their vegetarian digestive tracts.

How and why, then, did human beings begin eating flesh and animal products? Maybe we are truly omnivores who always ate small amounts of animal foods. But it also could be that we are truly vegetarians who were driven to consume animal foods in order to survive. In my opinion, natural disasters, drought being the most devastating, and migration to colder climates were probably the two major reasons that human beings began to incorporate animal foods into their diet. Suffering from hunger and faced with starvation, primitive people were forced to mimic omnivores and carnivores. Flesh, bird or snake eggs, or the milk of another species were better than death and extinction. Also, the lack of a mother's milk for her hungry infant surely resulted in the primitive people's domestication of other lactating species for infant food. I'm certain that only hunger due to drought would force mature adults to consume a food (milk) that is intended for another creature's young. Based on the type of digestive tract we have and on the fact that there are healthy, long-time, 100 percent vegetarians, I believe we were biologically intended to be vegetarian, but disastrous circumstances forced human beings to eat as omnivores.

What made primitive people continue to eat flesh and other animal foods? Surely the unconscious desire to fatten up in case of another drought played an important role. Cravings for foods that do not produce optimum health but satisfy the taste buds also helped perpetuate excessive consumption of animal foods. Similar cravings for foods that do not produce optimum health, sanctioned and promoted by governments, doctors, industry and advertising, keep millions of people in modern, industrialized societies and in Third World nations consuming concentrated, nutritionally deficient foods such as chocolate, soda, coffee, sugar, salt, fried foods, and refined foods. It is important to note that protein is a concentrated food and, like all of the above concentrated foods, produces a cyclical craving for more and more of the same and for other concentrated foods.

Religious rites and sacrifices also encouraged primitive people to continue eating flesh. Many primitive people believed that sacrificing an animal would please or appease the gods. Some also believed they could capture an animal's soul or strengths by devouring its flesh. These beliefs are not so unlike those of modern men in America who believe that eating beefsteaks will make them into strong and hardy cowboys or build Herculean bodies. More than likely, eating beefsteaks will give men breasts, fatten their thighs and rump, cause acne, make abdominal muscles sag, and hasten death.

And finally let's not forget profit. Owning animals and using their food by-products gave primitive people a leading edge when it came time to barter or sell. Individuals as well as communities could profit from the domestication and use of animals just as factory farmers and neighboring towns profit from animal agriculture in this century. Survival of the fittest has encouraged human beings to eat and use animals in any way we see fit, even if in the long run it is to the detriment of our health, the health of others, and the ecology.

The time has come, however, to leave rituals, habit, and profit behind and to abandon unhealthy food cravings. You can experience optimum health by becoming a vegetarian or eating a diet as close to vegetarianism as possible. Remember, the reduction of animal-food consumption by 70 percent, 80 percent, or 90 percent will have a tremendously positive influence on your health and longevity, not to mention what it will do for world hunger, the ecology, and animal suffering.

THE FOODS YOU DON'T EAT CAN HELP ELIMINATE MANY INJUSTICES

The elimination or significant reduction in the consumption of flesh foods, other animal products, and refined foods can do much more than improve your health. You can, by improving your diet, directly and indirectly, have a positive impact on the following issues:

1) World hunger and starvation
2) Ecological destruction
3) Animal suffering

Chances are you're not consciously aware of how eating animal foods affects these issues. You may have read and seen news reports about these topics, but you probably automatically block this information from your consciousness. These topics are too painful to confront. You try to bury these issues and your fears, as our society tries to bury its nuclear waste, but it doesn't work. They always return to haunt you. Helplessness and hopelessness prevail, and you sink into inertia and inactivity. You secretly hope somehow these problems will be resolved, but they won't, not without your help. It's up to each one of us to instigate the preliminary, grass roots actions that will pave the way for the changes that worldwide governments must make in order to eliminate world hunger, starvation, pollution, and animal abuse. Because governments and industries will never voluntarily take action we must push them. Your eating whole foods and foods that are lower on the food chain will gradually reduce the demand for flesh food, other animal products, and refined foods. The suppliers will have to reduce production and gradually shift to more sane, ethical, and ecologically safe income-producing businesses.

Major industries in the United States have already begun to develop new products (whole-grain breads and breakfast cereals are now available in supermarkets from major producers) in response to consumer demand. Governments worldwide will ease the transition within their own country by giving farmers subsidies (Canada is now subsidizing organic farmers), and you will know that your actions (dietary changes) were responsible for beginning a momentum toward a better world.

Starvation and World Hunger

Starvation and world hunger are two separate issues requiring our attention and action. Starvation occurs mostly in Third World nations. Starvation means to die from lack of food or nourishment. I know you think no one should starve to death. I also know you think there is nothing you can do about it. You are wrong. If Americans would reduce meat consumption by only 10 percent, enough soybeans and grains would become available to save 60 million people a year from starving to death. This is because every pound of flesh food requires 14 pounds of grain to produce it. If humans ate the grain directly, it would spread available foods 14 times further! You can make a personal commitment to the 60 million people who die annually of starvation by reducing your personal intake of animal flesh and other animal foods. Don't do it and keep your mouth shut about it. Tell your friends, acquaintances, and business associates. Write letters to key politicians and to the president of your country, telling them you are reducing your consumption of animal foods and why. Imagine the impact if Americans and concerned citizens in countries worldwide decided to reduce their consumption of animal foods by 70 percent, 80 percent, or 90 percent as a personal statement regarding starvation. Gestures of this nature would attract the attention of our world leaders and force them into action.

Hunger generally refers to the lack of sufficient food to fill the stomach; it can also refer to the absence of the right kinds of foods in a full stomach—foods that supply the nutrients needed by the body to maintain optimum health. There are hungry people in modern, industrialized nations as well as in Third World nations. Hunger caused by a lack of food can be remedied by providing the needed foods. Proper and sane food management on a worldwide scale can make this possible. The phenomenon of hunger with a full stomach exists because most people consume empty carbohydrates (refined grain foods), overcooked (fiber- and nutrient-deficient) vegetables, insufficient amounts of fresh fruits, and excessive quantities of animal-protein foods devoid of fiber. Hunger caused by consuming the wrong kinds of foods can also be eliminated by educating people and by providing the appropriate foods. If the body does not receive the nutrients required from the food consumed, it will continually demand more food as it seeks the missing nutrients. This is one of many reasons why people overeat.

Eating inappropriate foods can also cause the body to lose completely the desire for health-giving foods and crave only junk foods. These foods artificially stimulate the body and disguise the underlying need for the nutrients it requires. Junk foods create another kind of hunger; a cyclical hunger for more of the same junk foods. Most of us living in modern, civilized nations do not experience starvation or hunger due to a lack of food. We usually have enough or more than enough food to eat. Our problem is educating ourselves to eat foods that encourage optimum health, discourage world hunger and starvation, favor a sane ecology, and eliminate animal suffering. In sympathy for those people who starve to death annually and as a political statement, consider becoming a vegetarian or reducing your consumption of animal foods and refined processed foods.

The unavailability of food is not the primary cause of hunger or starvation. Some experts say there is already enough grain to feed every human being on this planet. Others say that if all the grains in the world currently being fed to farm animals were properly directed to those people who are hungry and starving, this injustice would be well on its way to a resolution. If all the grains currently being held off the market, burned, allowed to rot, or shipped to the upper classes of Third World nations were also redirected, we would have more than we need to feed every hungry human being on this planet. Most people simply do not realize that giving up certain foods or eating less of these foods can make a difference to the world hunger situation. It will make a difference, perhaps not for this generation of hungry and starving people but surely for future generations.

If our political leaders and other authority figures, worldwide, would move toward adopting and advocating a vegetarian lifestyle and philosophy, both world hunger and starvation would one day cease to exist. All people worldwide would have ample unrefined grains, fresh vegetables, fresh fruit, legumes, raw seeds, and raw nuts. If life on this planet is to continue in a sane manner, we need world leaders who are prepared to change to a life-preserving, conservation-oriented lifestyle and philosophy. We also need you and everyone else to participate and initiate the necessary changes.

The organization listed below can lead you to more literature on this subject:

FOOD FIRST
The Institute for Food and Development Policy
2588 Mission Street
San Francisco, CA 94110

Destruction of Our Planet by Animal Husbandry

Pollution and ecological destruction of our planet is now so great that, according to some experts, it may already be too late to reverse their effects. Animal agribusiness contributes to the ecological destruction of our planet in many ways. Most of us believe animal manure replenishes needed nutrients to the soil. This used to be so, but now we are raising too many animals resulting in too much animal excrement. Manure is poisoning our soil, offsetting the natural chemical balance of the soil, contributing to the greenhouse effect, and polluting our ground water. Our already depleted water supply is being further threatened by the wasteful use of water in the factory-farm industries. It's hard to believe, but one pound of beefsteak wastes 2500 gallons of water and 50 out of every 100 gallons of non-recyclable water are wasted on the irrigation of livestock grains. The dairy industry is also wasting enormous amounts of water. It is difficult to believe, but 100 gallons of water is used (wasted) to produce one pat of butter. This waste must stop before it's too late.

Because of animal farming, one-third of the topsoil in our major farming areas has been eroded and half of the tropical rain forests of South America have been cut down to provide grazing land for American cattle raisers. The latter is having a disastrous effect on our ecology. The carbon dioxide buildup from the burning and cutting of these trees is accelerating the greenhouse effect, which could sufficiently melt the polar ice caps to flood the coastal cities and lowlands. Deforestation is also responsible for the extinction and death of thousands of species of animals, birds, reptiles, insects, flowers, herbs, etc. The consumption of excessive amounts of animal foods is destroying our planet in too many ways to discuss in this book. Please learn more, and begin to modify your diet so you can live your beliefs while getting healthier.

The following books discuss animal husbandry and its detrimental effect on our ecology.

DIET FOR A NEW AMERICA
John Robbins
Stillpoint Publishing
Box 640
Meeting House Road
Walpole, NH 03608
1-800-847-4041

ANIMAL FACTORIES
Jim Mason and Peter Singer
The Animals Agenda
P.O. Box 5234
Westport, CT 06881

FOOD REFORM: OUR DESPERATE NEED
Robin Hur
Progressive Products
P.O. Box 333
Amherst, MA 01004

ANIMAL LIBERATION
Peter Singer
Avon Books
1790 Broadway
New York, NY 10019

DIET FOR A SMALL PLANET
10th Anniversary Edition
Frances Moore Lappe
Ballantine Books
201 East 50th Street
New York, N.Y.
(212) 751-2600

HOOF PRINTS ON THE FOREST
Available from the U.S. government Printing Office
Retail Book Store
26 Federal Plaza
New York, NY
(212) 264-3826

A STUDY ON CENTRAL AMERICA
Available from the U.S. government

DEEP ECOLOGY
Bill Devall and George Sessions

SACRED COWS AT THE PUBLIC TROUGH
Denzil and Nancy Ferguson

The last two books may be purchased from:
EARTH FIRST!
P.O. Box 5871
Tuscon, AZ 85703

Animal Suffering

The inhumane treatment of the animals that provide flesh, eggs, and dairy products is another tragic problem that can be resolved by eating foods that are lower on the food chain or by adopting a vegetarian diet. Rarely do farm animals graze lazily in sunny fields. Indeed, most farm animals live out their lives in misery, confinement, isolation, and deprivation until they are led to their inevitable, terrifying slaughter. If you think animals don't know fear, go to a slaughterhouse and witness the terror and panic for yourself. Up until that final, terrifying moment, most factory-farm animals never see the light of day, experience a fresh breeze, or feel the earth beneath their feet. Most of them are constantly flooded with harsh, bright, artificial light or, at the other extreme, forced to live 22 hours a day in total darkness. They lie or stand on cold, concrete floors or, much worse, wire floors that cripple their hoofs or claws. This can hardly be called humane treatment.

I am sure you do not approve of animal suffering and that you do not want to participate in this uncivilized method of raising farm animals. But you are, each time you eat flesh foods or other animal products. What you see on your plate has not magically materialized. Feeling, sentient creatures have suffered *horribly* for your every mouthful.

No farm animal is excluded from this inhumane treatment, not even the intelligent pig. Their intelligence is similar to that of dogs. Pigs are faithful, curious, playful, friendly, sociable, and feeling creatures. Pigs, by nature, are very clean animals. They live in mud and their own excrement only because confinement forces them to do so. A factory farm sow spends her life pregnant and in confinement, her stall so small that it is impossible for her to turn around. When labor begins, she is immobilized by a device in which she is forced to remain until her young are weaned; then she is once again impregnated and returned to her confining stall to repeat the cycle, a cycle that will be repeated again and again until her slaughter. No animal should be treated in such a manner.

Calves, too, are confined to stalls, but calves have even less space for movement than pigs; calves haven't even enough room to lie down comfortably. Calves are taken from their mothers at birth and fed a ration that intentionally makes them anemic. They live in a covered wooden crate that's too small for movement and spend at least 22 hours a day in total darkness. Is any veal dinner—no matter how tender—worth all this suffering and deprivation?

Dairy cattle no longer roam idly on lush green pasture lands. A dairy cow knows no joy. She usually spends her entire life in one or two over-crowded buildings, where chemicals are administered to force her to produce more milk than she is naturally able to produce. Many cows collapse from exhaustion, and, when they do, no time is wasted on treatment or care. Instead, they are immediately shipped to a slaughterhouse. If a cow is too exhausted to walk through the doorway, she is electrically prodded to force her to walk across the threshold of the slaughterhouse. There is a financial "justification" for this electrical prodding: A cow that can walk across the slaughterhouse doorway is worth more per pound than one that can't. Not only is this unfair and inhumane treatment, but, from the perspective of your health, this totally exhausted creature is hardly fit for human consumption. Any cow whose milk production falls below the acceptable level shares the same fate. Kosher cows are even more unfortunate when it comes to their slaughter. They are hoisted up by one leg and left dangling on a conveyer system, sometimes for as long as ten minutes, until their throats are slit. Try to imagine the pain a cow weighing several hundred pounds must experience while hanging by one leg for even one minute. These unfortunate creatures cannot possibly be providing healthy milk for you and your children, and undoubtedly their flesh can only be termed "sick meat." A cow is producing milk for her baby calf, and her flesh is not what our long vegetarian digestive tracts are meant to consume. Reconsider your present eating habits. Are you certain you want to continue eating "sick meat" and drinking the "milk of misery"?

Of all farm animals, chickens fare the worst. Very few people have sympathy for chickens; we assume they are stupid creatures. A local farmer I knew as a child taught me to believe that too. I once met a pet chicken—a friendly, curious, intelligent creature. My experience with this chicken showed me that chickens have endearing qualities like other animals. She would have changed your opinion too.

Factory-farm conditions crowd up to nine chickens into a cage measuring *18 by 24 inches*; only the death of a few birds in a cage (a circumstance that is inevitable because of the overcrowding) affords the remaining chickens additional space. No veterinary treatment is provided for injured or sick birds. Their claws often grow so long that they grow around the wire floors, thus immobilizing the birds until their death. Chickens are so frustrated by the overcrowding that their beaks have to be burned so they do not peck each other to death. Finally, these tortured, miserable creatures are hung upside down and moved along a conveyor to their terrifying slaughter. No creature deserves such treatment.

Consider the inhumane circumstances that the factory farm imposes upon animals. Do you want to contribute to this? If you are an animal lover, you surely don't. Perhaps you don't *love* animals; even so, do you believe we are free to inflict such suffering? If you are not moved by the suffering of these animals, think about yourself. These creatures are not in good health; you cannot possibly obtain optimum health by eating stagnant, overfed, drugged, confined, miserable, terrified, distressed, sick animals. If you don't care about your health, consider the health of your children and other people's children who unknowingly consume the flesh and by-products of these unfortunate, sick animals. I know at least one of the above atrocities has meaning for you. Don't block it. Change your diet. You *can* make a difference!

The following books will tell you more. *Be brave!* Read. If what you read makes you cry, scream and lose your appetite, take action, become a vegetarian or eat low on the food chain as often as you can. The animals have no voice. They need your voice!

DIET FOR A NEW AMERICA
John Robbins
Stillpoint Publishing
Box 640
Meeting House Road
Walpole, NH 03608
1-800-847-4041

THE EXTENDED CIRCLE
Jon Wynne-Tyson
The International Society for Animal Rights
421 South State Street
Clarks Summit, PA 18411

FETTERED KINGDOMS
John Bryant
People for the Ethical Treatment of Animals
P.O. Box 42516
Washington, D.C. 20015

ANIMAL LIBERATION
Peter Singer
Avon Books
1790 Broadway
New York, NY 10019

ANIMALS, NATURE & ALBERT SCHWEITZER
Ann Cottrell Free, Editor
The Albert Schweitzer Fellowship
866 United Nations Plaza
New York, NY 10017

THE CASE FOR ANIMAL RIGHTS
Tom Regan
University of California Press
Berkeley, CA 94720

IN DEFENSE OF ANIMALS
Peter Singer, Editor
Basil Blackwell Inc.
432 Park Avenue South, Suite 1505
New York, NY 10016

Purchase the last two books from:

The Animals Agenda
P.O. Box 5234
Westport, CT 06881

WHAT WE EAT AND WHY WE EAT IT

My childhood meals were typical of those shared by most Canadian and American families. Each meal was centered around animal protein. Usually there were eggs, bacon, milk, and toast with jam for breakfast; a sandwich with iceberg lettuce and cheese or processed meat, milk, and an apple for lunch; and red meat or chicken or occasionally fish, potatoes, and a vegetable for dinner. Potatoes and/or white bread or some other refined carbohydrates (Quaker Oats was probably the least refined grain I consumed) accompanied the animal protein, while vegetables (usually canned or frozen, but sometimes fresh and almost always overcooked) were relegated to the role of providing "color contrast." Salads consisted of iceberg lettuce, cucumbers, and tomatoes. Most meals were followed by a refined sugar-sweet dessert or by canned fruit. Baked desserts, homemade or store-bought, usually won in popularity over fresh fruit. Salt was in most foods I ate.

As you can gather, I came from a rather typical gastronomical background. I did not emerge from a nutritionally enlightened family who helped pioneer the practice of eating whole-grain, unprocessed foods or vegetarian fare. In spite of it all, I've been able to totally change the way I eat, and I don't feel the least bit deprived. In fact, I am rarely tempted by the foods I used to eat.

For the most part, my dietary changes evolved slowly over the years, although there were periods of rapid and sudden enlightenment and change. My new eating patterns have more than rewarded me with abundant energy and improved health as well as the knowledge that I am not indirectly contributing to world hunger and starvation or directly contributing to the destruction of the ecology of our planet and to the suffering of animals.

To help you understand which foods to consume for optimum health, I must first explain why we eat what we eat. Once you have a clear picture of the motivations behind your eating habits, you can more easily consider implementing the necessary changes that will lead to your optimum health.

PERSONAL PREFERENCES

Personal preferences for particular foods usually stem from infancy or early childhood. If your mother fed you fruit foods before vegetable foods, she may have unknowingly set up a preference for sweet-tasting foods so that you now dislike vegetables. Food preferences are also quite often linked with an early positive or negative emotional experience. The mood of the child or the mother can determine how the child reacts to a newly introduced food. A tired or upset mother is less likely to introduce a new food with great enthusiasm, especially if she is in a bad mood. Positive communication, verbal or nonverbal, makes infants and children more receptive to new foods. Infants have a natural instinct for wholesome foods, but this can be thwarted if a food is introduced in a negative atmosphere or manner. Unpleasant emotions experienced at the time of introducing a new food can produce an aversion to that food even if it is a wholesome food. A child will often retain an aversion for a particular food into adult life even though the food is known to be beneficial for his or her health.

Become an adventurer. Try foods that promote optimum health. Allow yourself time to acquire a taste for a new food. Initially, try at least three unbiased mouthfuls. Then, a week or so apart, allow yourself at least three or four different samplings of this food. Then decide if this food is going to become part of your new diet. Chances are you'll find you will be able to adapt to many new tastes using this technique, and even the foods that taste bizarre initially will quite possibly become your favorites.

CULTURAL PREFERENCES

Cultural food preferences are acquired from our parents and immediate family. For example, a mother may love sausage because she is Italian and her mother loved sausage; so when she puts the sausage in her child's mouth she says, "Umm! This is good, sweetheart!" The response will probably be favorable, even though the child's taste buds find the sausage unappealing. Likewise, family gatherings and festive holidays form cultural food preferences. If ham was traditional fare at your family Christmas dinner, now, as an adult, you may simply not be able to imagine Christmas without it, although you never eat ham at any other time of the year because you find it too salty.

Cultural food preferences keep your mind and taste buds unresponsive to new and wonderful taste sensations. Sample unfamiliar, health-promoting foods with curiosity and enthusiasm, not with a closed mind. Sometimes it takes weeks or months to appreciate a new taste sensation. I've had patients and friends try seaweed or raw sesame tahini with varying responses. Some people love these foods immediately. Their bodies seem to know it's nutritious. Other people take weeks or months to acquire a taste for seaweed or sesame tahini. Be brave; persist and you will conquer your cultural prejudices against new foods.

INCOME

Your financial situation often determines what you will or will not eat. All too often people say that organic food is too expensive. Good food that promotes optimum health is never too expensive. The same people who object to the high cost of health-promoting foods eat expensive pastries, cakes, cookies; smoke cigarettes; and drink liquor or soda—all without a thought for the money they are wasting. They also do not consider the eventual dental bills they will pay to repair their rotting teeth. Nor do they consider the cost of medical treatment for diseases they acquire by consuming these nonnutritive foods and beverages. The cost of organic foods is rarely the only reason why a person won't healthfully feed their body. Sometimes a person feels they don't deserve the best foods because they secretly believe they don't deserve to be healthy and happy. Everyone deserves to be healthy and happy. Buying inferior foods rarely gives you the oral satisfaction you seek or the nutrition you require. Think about it. Do you believe you do not deserve the best foods? If so, break your negative programming. Your health will flourish, and the ecology will benefit because foods grown organically nourish the earth and do not contribute billions of tons of toxic chemicals annually to our soil and ground water. Finally, consider the extra money spent on organic food as an investment in your health, an investment in a positive-impact industry, and an investment in your planet.

TIME SCHEDULE

Do you feel you have only enough time to grab a hot dog or a hamburger? If you are constantly on the go and away from home, it may seem easier to settle for less health-supporting foods, but *with a little planning* you can easily make quick, nutritious snacks. Prepare three different types of grains twice a week, and store them in the refrigerator. Take a portion or two along with you each day that you are away from home. If you don't have time to prepare a salad or cook some vegetables to eat with your grain, don't give up. Neighborhood health-food stores, fresh-vegetable markets, and supermarkets sell string beans, snow peas, alfalfa sprouts, watercress, etc., any of which you can eat raw with your grain. Fresh fruit, raw seeds, and raw nuts are also available in almost every food store for a quick, nutritious, delicious, and inexpensive snack. If you are not on a budget, locate a health-food restaurant or two in your neighborhood; it can become your new, favorite lunch spot. Eat small snacks when you are away from home or when you don't have time to cook. Save the heartier meals for when you have the time to prepare them and the time to eat them.

ADVERTISING CAMPAIGNS

Advertising is perhaps one of the most subtle and convincing methods of developing food preferences. Major food industries spend billions of dollars annually to convince you that their products are good tasting and good for your health, though many of them have been proven not to be the latter. Most of us fall victim to these large advertising campaigns. You probably have too. Free yourself from this form of brainwashing that keeps these multibillion-dollar industries thriving. Adopt a health-promoting diet. Eat low on the food chain as often as you can, or become a vegetarian. For further information and guidance on foods for optimum health or vegetarianism, read Dr. John A. McDougall's two books, *The McDougall Plan* and *McDougall Medicine*, as well as the two cookbooks by his wife Mary McDougall. These books are, in my opinion, among the best available.

Carefully consider all of the above five reasons why you eat what you eat; discover which of these traps you have fallen into. Break free! Learn to enjoy and crave those foods that will enable you to obtain and maintain optimum health.

FLESH AND ANIMAL FOODS DO NOT PROMOTE OPTIMUM HEALTH

The majority of people have come to accept as fact several false notions about vegetarianism. These misconceptions are because of a previous lack of medical information on the subject, the attempts of government and industry to convince us that animal protein is essential for optimum health, and unintentional misinformation that has been passed on orally and in print.

Students in elementary school, high school, and college are taught that the four basic food groups are precisely what must be eaten for sound health. Required are two or more servings daily from the meat group, which includes red meat, chicken, fish, eggs, and legumes, or in other words, "protein"; three or more servings from the milk group, which includes milk and all kinds of cheeses as well as ice cream, or once again, "protein"; four or more servings of vegetables and fruits from the third group; and finally, from the fourth group, four or more servings of breads and cereals (unfortunately, the posters usually illustrate refined breads and cereals, not whole-grain products).

Let's look more closely at these four basic food groups. How were these food requirements determined in the first place? Animal experiments funded by the government and/or major industries have been the most accepted methods of determining the nutritional requirements of human beings. Many reputable scientists now openly state that animal experiments are cruel and useless because the results obtained from one species rarely apply to another species. Each species has its own nutritional requirements.

For example, the milk protein required by growing infant rats is ten times greater than that required by a human infant. Adult rats require as much as three and a half times more protein than an adult human. Why, then, were rats used to determine our nutritional needs? One reason is that it is cheaper to experiment on rats than on human beings. Another is that the protein-supplying industries want us to believe we require a greater, rather than a lesser, amount of protein because it suits their profit-making goals. The original animal experiments conducted in 1914 by Osborn and Mendel to determine human protein needs were done on rats. Osborn and Mendel discovered that rats grew better on animal protein than they did on vegetable protein, thereby leading to the erroneous conclusion that vegetable protein is incomplete and unsatisfactory for people who want to obtain optimum health.

In the 1940s, William Rose published that ten amino acids were essential for a rat's diet. This experiment seemed to confirm that grains and vegetables are incomplete foods and deficient in amino acids that human beings require for optimum health. The saga of amino acid requirements continued until 1952, when William Rose, by testing human beings, determined that only eight (not ten) amino acids were truly essential for adult human beings. Recent evidence proves that plant amino acid patterns are ideal for optimum human health. Two amino acids, arginine and histidine, are additionally required by infants; they are available in mother's milk. If a mother is unable to provide enough milk, the best substitutes are a wet nurse or human milk obtained from a milk bank. After the age of four most people naturally lose the ability to efficiently digest the carbohydrate known as lactose, which is one reason why it is better for adults not to consume dairy products. Allergic reactions, high protein, high fat and cholesterol content are three more excellent reasons why dairy products are not ideal for human consumption.

Studies indicate that Seventh-Day Adventists (children and adults) thrive on a vegetarian diet consisting of whole grains, assorted vegetables, fruits, legumes, seeds, and nuts. Other studies indicate that when our modern Western diet infiltrates into nonindustrialized nations, health in those nations significantly decreases. For further information on this subject, read Dr. McDougall's books and *Diet for a Small Planet*, which are listed in the bibliography.

Another important question to ask in this matter is: Who is sponsoring the printing and distribution of the charts illustrating these four basic food groups? Look closely at the small print on these beautifully illustrated and convincingly designed charts; you will discover that they are distributed by the four major food industries as self-serving advertisements for their own food products. These charts do not accurately reflect our true nutritional needs. The government subsidizes the food industries, and the medical establishment allows them to advertise in their journals, which further promulgates this dietary misinformation while pharmaceutical companies annually make a tremendous profit on the drugs we "need" to control the symptoms of the diseases we acquire from our incorrect diets. This cycle must end. You can improve your health and help to end all the injustices that accompany the animal-farming industries by gradually reducing your consumption of these foods or by becoming a pure vegetarian.

COMMON MISCONCEPTIONS ABOUT VEGETARIANISM

THE FEAR OF PROTEIN DEPRIVATION

Most people in industrialized nations are convinced they require three or four servings of animal protein daily. If this quota is not met, they believe their hair will fall out, their nails will break, their skin will become diseased, and, ultimately, their vigor and stamina will be reduced to a point near death. Certainly, we do need adequate amounts of protein but not nearly as much as we have been led to believe—and the protein need not come from animal sources. Sufficient lit-

erature exists to establish that plant protein is *totally adequate* for human protein requirements. Legumes, raw seeds, raw nuts, grains, vegetables, and fruit all contain the amino acids we require. In fact, legumes, raw seeds, and raw nuts contain such high amounts of protein (amino acids) and oils that their consumption must, in some cases, be restricted. It is entirely possible to obtain too much protein or oil from plant sources. Excess protein, whether from animal or plant sources, is broken down in the liver and is excreted via the kidneys. Along with this protein waste, i.e., blood urea nitrogen, the kidneys also excrete many minerals, including calcium. This is due to the diuretic nature of urea. High-protein diets, therefore, create a negative calcium balance in the body, even if the calcium intake is very high.

One of the many results of a high-protein diet is osteoporosis, which afflicts many women in their senior years. Worldwide observations of populations that do not consume high quantities of animal protein show that osteoporosis is almost nonexistent.

Our rich, modern diet not only causes mineral loss; it also causes kidney disease by progressively destroying kidney tissue. Purines, usually abundant in high-protein foods, become uric acid and accumulate in the joints causing gouty arthritis. Purines also form uric acid kidney stones in some people. Animal protein has no fiber and is low in carbohydrates and potassium, all of which are essential for optimum health. Flesh foods and other animal products are high in sodium, fat, and cholesterol. It has been well established that fat and cholesterol cause a number of illnesses and, consequently, a great deal of suffering. Another important factor to remember is that flesh and other animal products are extremely high in livestock chemicals as well as environmental contaminants. Both categories of toxins are extremely detrimental to our systems and are suspected of causing cancer, birth defects, and other toxic reactions.

EXCELLENT SOURCES OF VEGETARIAN CALCIUM

Perhaps one of the greatest fears is that adequate calcium cannot be obtained on a totally vegetarian diet. This is absolutely *not* true. If you consume dark-green vegetables three times daily, you will definitely get all the calcium you require. In fact, as the chart below, adapted from Dr. Agatha Thrash's book, *Eat For Strength* (Thrash Publications, Route 1, Box 273, Seale, AL 36875), shows, many vegetarian foods supply as much or more calcium than milk.

Other vegetables, as well as grains, raw seeds, raw nuts, legumes, and fruit, all contain calcium. To reassure yourself, remember that in many parts of the world where dairy products are not eaten, calcium deficiencies have rarely been found. Western vegetarian societies do not have calcium deficiencies either. The body is much more efficient than we realize. If the dietary calcium is low, the body absorbs more from our foods than it would if we were consuming high dietary levels of calcium. It is also important to remember that dairy foods are high in protein, and high-protein foods cause the loss of calcium in the urine. In fact, doctors specializing in vegetarian nutrition say that the calcium RDA, 1200 mg., may only be necessary for people on high protein diets (e.g., the average American diet). Vegetarians consume less protein and therefore need less calcium than the RDA. Also of interest is the fact that low-fat dairy products, which many people consume, do not favor the assimilation of calcium. Fat actually aids in the assimilation of calcium. The body more easily obtains its calcium from snacks and meals low in concentrated protein. Too much vegetarian protein (legumes, raw seeds, raw nuts, etc.) can also cause calcium loss. Ultimately, consuming less protein is better for your health because not only do you lose calcium on a high-protein diet but you also lose other minerals. Minerals are very important for achieving and maintaining optimum health.

THE VITAMIN B_{12} CONTROVERSY

A vitamin B_{12} deficiency can be very serious, even potentially fatal, and is a major concern of prospective vegetarians. Extreme fatigue, confusion, disorientation, deterioration of the nervous system, menstrual disturbances, difficulty in walking, and brain damage are some of the many symptoms associated with vitamin B_{12} deficiencies. Because there is controversy surrounding the adequacy of a purely vegetarian diet, it is imperative *you* feel confident that vitamin B_{12} can be obtained from a nonanimal source or, at the very least, from a supplement. Vegetarian sources of this vitamin are controversial, yet only rarely are vitamin B_{12} deficiencies due to an inadequate diet. In fact, the vast majority of vitamin B_{12} deficiencies are due to pernicious anemia, a disease

COMPARISON OF SOME SOURCES OF CALCIUM

Food	Quantity	Grams
Collards	1 cup	.498 grams
Dandelions	1 cup	.336 grams
Mustard Greens	¾ cup	.330 grams
Cooked Turnip Greens	¾ cup	.304 grams
Milk	*1 cup*	*.283 grams*
Kale	1 cup	.248 grams
Broccoli	1 cup	.245 grams
Cooked Beans	1 cup	.146 grams
Dried figs	4 figs	.134 grams
Blackstrap Molasses	1 Tbsp	.116 grams

that involves the body's inability to properly absorb this nutrient.

Doctors, scientists, and authors of government literature tell us that vitamin B_{12} is only obtainable from animal sources. How then do 100 percent pure vegetarians, who do not consume animal products or vitamin B_{12} supplements, remain healthy? Research indicates some plant foods such as spirulina and fermented, unpasteurized foods (tofu, tempeh, raw sauerkraut, etc.) supply small amounts of vitamin B_{12}. However, they also supply an analogue (false) vitamin B_{12}. There is some speculation that these analogues may block the assimilation of true vitamin B_{12}, but this has not been conclusively proven for human beings. So, perhaps, 100 percent pure vegetarians are obtaining some vitamin B_{12} from these foods.

The dietary requirement for vitamin B_{12} is so small (one millionth of a gram) and it is stored so well in the body that people may be able to obtain all the vitamin B_{12} they require from vitamin B_{12}-producing bacteria in their mouths and intestines. In fact, vitamin B_{12}-producing microorganisms are everywhere: on your hands, in the air, on your dinner plate, and on the fruits and vegetables you eat. Excessive cleaning of fruits and vegetables, which many people do in the hope of removing the chemicals with which they are sprayed, washes away one of the easiest to obtain sources of vitamin B_{12}. Similarly, antibiotics, medications, and alcohol and other recreational drugs will destroy systemic vitamin B_{12}-producing bacteria. Therefore, if you have a history of drug taking, you will not be able to count on this bacterial source.

If you choose not to consume animal sources of this nutrient and feel uncertain about bacterial sources, taking supplemental vitamin B_{12} can be viewed as optional insurance, even though many healthy, long-term vegetarians have never taken vitamin B_{12} supplements. Vitamin B_{12} can be obtained either by supplementing your diet with vitamin B_{12} injections, by utilizing nasal vitamin B_{12}, or by taking sublingual vitamin B_{12}. If you want to take vitamin B_{12} as a supplement, the nasal form, now available in health-food stores, assimilates better than sublingual tablets. The nasal form of vitamin B_{12} is so easily assimilated through the nasal membrane that it is almost as reliable a source as a vitamin B_{12} injection. Inconclusive studies seem to indicate that vitamin B_{12} in ordinary tablet form has an antivitamin B_{12} effect in the system and can cause a deficiency of vitamin B_{12} even if your diet is adequate. If the reports of these studies leave you feeling uncertain, avoid vitamin B_{12} tablets, vitamin B complex formulas, or any multiple vitamin and mineral supplements containing vitamin B_{12}.

Given how low our need for vitamin B_{12} is, if you plan to reduce your animal-protein intake to two servings per week, you probably do not need to worry about meeting your vitamin B_{12} requirements. It is important to note that there is a lot of controversy on the vitamin B_{12} issue, so read up on this subject. You must feel comfortable with your decision regarding the supplementation of vitamin B_{12}. There are several medical doctors who have written on the vitamin B_{12} issue and stated that supplementing vitamin B_{12} is not absolutely necessary. Consult Dr. McDougall's books and Dr. Klapper's books.

AMINO ACID COMPLEMENTING IS COMPLICATED AND UNNECESSARY

Another common misconception about vegetarianism and protein requirements is that it is impossible to obtain the proper balance of amino acids from purely vegetarian sources unless you embark on a complicated system of amino acid complementing to balance the amino acids of, for example, grains with those of legumes. The original research that led to this erroneous conclusion was based on early experiments with rats, which took for granted that we require as much protein as rats and that it was necessary for human beings to consume an amino acid balance similar to that provided by animal foods. But we do not require nearly as much protein as rats, and we do not have to complement amino acids in order to create similar or identical amino acid patterns. Frances Moore Lappe's revolutionary book, *Diet for a Small Planet*, published in 1972, originally recommended amino acid complementing to assure her readers a vegetarian diet would provide complete protein. Rat-protein research data was the basis for her recommendations. She now views amino acid complementing as unnecessary, and this is reflected in the revised tenth anniversary edition of her book.

It is even possible to obtain too much vegetarian protein. Legumes (beans, peas, lentils, peanuts, etc.) are high in vegetarian protein, and their consumption should be limited. If you are already in optimum health, *up to* one cup of legumes is permissible per day. If you wish to improve your health, consume less or no legumes until you reach the desired results. Raw seeds and raw nuts are also high in protein. If you consume legumes, raw seeds, or raw nuts in one day, be certain to reduce the amount of legumes you eat to allow for the added protein offered by the raw seeds and raw nuts. Also, do not eat too many raw nuts or raw seeds each day. More than two to four tablespoons of raw-nut or raw-seed butter each day may be too much for some people. Do not worry about complementing your amino acids in grains and legumes. If you eat whole foods low on the food chain, you will have no problems with protein deficiencies.

A PROGRAM FOR OPTIMUM HEALTH

Perhaps you are now ready to embark on your new dietary program. Please read what follows carefully, and reread it several times. It is easy to become confused and misinterpret information; a lot is presented at once. Do not feel compelled to change your diet overnight, unless, of course, it feels right to make a radical change. My dietary conclusions have evolved over a period of ten years. Personal experimentation, research, and observation have led me to believe that the closer your diet is to total vegetarianism the healthier you will be.

Don't ever feel that you *must* make dietary changes. Modify your diet because you are fed up with feeling sick, pain, fatigue, etc., or because you are concerned with the prevention of disease

and premature aging. Modify your diet because you *want* to feel better and look better. The process of improving your diet is an adventure you will enjoy because *you* made the choice to experience optimum health and *you* made the choice to have a positive impact on global issues. Make changes at your own pace. Gradual modifications are easier to cope with and are less of a shock to your body and mind. Don't get discouraged and give up if you temporarily slip back into your old eating habits; simply get back to living your beliefs as soon as you are able. It is perfectly natural to return to foods you once craved or enjoyed. Emotionally, you need to feel and know that you are not trapped, restricted, or denied. If you feel you can *never* have a particular food, you will, like most people, feel rebellious. If you know you can have it but are *choosing* to have it less frequently, on special occasions, or when you really, really need it, you will feel in control and peaceful with your decision. With the passage of time you will comfortably begin to lose your desire for many or most of the unhealthy foods you once cherished. You will be satisfied with having these foods infrequently. New desires and a craving for healthy foods will develop.

For greater detail, precise statistics, and thoroughly documented books on vegetarianism, please read Dr. John McDougall and Mary McDougall's books, *The McDougall Plan*, *McDougall Medicine* and *The McDougall Health Supporting Cookbook*. I was thrilled to discover these books. They provided me with some of the missing links that have changed my personal beliefs and suspicions into trustworthy information. In addition, these books have given me great hope. We need more physicians to research thoroughly the available literature pertaining to vegetarianism. We need qualified, brave spokespersons who are willing to stand up for their convictions, even if it means going against tradition and the establishment. Dr. McDougall and his wife Mary are truly pioneers in the field of vegetarian nutrition. Fortunately, throughout history, determined individuals like the McDougalls have emerged ready to fight for what they know is right. Equally fortunately, there have always been large numbers of people ready, some more quickly than others, to accept new, convincing, and well-documented theories. I sincerely hope this chapter will interest you enough to encourage you to eagerly seek out the McDougalls' books, which will convince you, once and for all, that eating as close to vegetarianism as you possibly can is the only way to achieve optimum health, help eliminate world hunger and starvation, end animal suffering, and improve the ecology of the world.

Before you proceed, I have a few helpful hints to offer on how to eat.

- *Eat four to six "Snack-Meals" daily to maintain high energy levels.* Digestion draws blood from the brain to the digestive organs, leaving you with diminished mental abilities. To avoid this, eat smaller, more frequent meals ("snack-meals") instead of fewer, larger meals. If you eat in this manner, you will not feel sleepy after meals. You will also be much less likely to experience digestive disturbances.

- *Eat one food at a time.* If you have digestive difficulties, it is best to eat one food at a time. For example, for lunch you are eating four different foods, such as sesame brown rice, steamed broccoli and carrots, begin with the sesame rice (for oral gratification purposes, you may eat sesame rice as one food); eat it all and enjoy it. Then eat the next food, and then the last. This method of eating simplifies the messages to the brain regarding the foods that are on their way down, and the proper amounts of digestive juices are more likely to be available for digestion.

- *Pay attention to food-combining rules if you have poor digestion.* (Note that I am not referring here to amino acid complementing.) If you digest anything and everything and never have fatigue, gas, bloating, belching, or pain after eating, food combining is less important for you. If you experience any or all of the above symptoms, you may want to experiment with food combining. Buy a book or chart. The basic rules are:

    1) Eat one protein per meal.
    2) Vegetarian protein and desserts or fruits don't combine (though some people can digest fruits and raw nuts or raw seeds).
    3) Animal protein and fruit or desserts don't combine.
    4) Animal protein and starches (carbohydrates) don't combine.
    5) Protein and additional oils don't combine well (for example, seeds roasted in oil or nuts and oils added to already high-protein foods for cooking purposes).
    6) Carbohydrates and desserts or fruits don't combine well.
    7) Carbohydrates and oils don't digest well (though most people can digest grains with raw seed- or raw nut-butter sauces).
    8) Raw fruits and raw vegetables usually don't combine well.
    9) Avoid eating more than three different foods at one meal.

Food combining rules can be followed strictly, or you can learn with time and experimentation which rules apply best to your body.

- *Consume all oil-rich foods before 6 P.M.* Our digestive functions are more efficient before six o'clock. After six, body functions, especially digestion, begin a period of decreased activity. To avoid indigestion and fatigue, eat oil-rich foods for lunch or for an early dinner. Raw seeds, raw nuts, and avocados are rich in digestible, essential fatty acids. Bottled oils are not recommended as a source of essential fatty acids. Only flaxseed oil that has been processed at low temperatures free of light and oxygen and packed in totally opaque containers provides a healthy source of concentrated oils. I believe, however, that only uncooked, whole, oil-rich foods are a balanced way of getting your fatty acids.

- *Consume oil-rich foods first.* The body receives the first message of needed digestive juices better than subsequent messages. Because oil-rich foods are more difficult to digest, it is advisable to eat these foods first. It is also pleasant to finish a meal with a clean, light taste. For example, if you are eating buckwheat noodles with a sesame tahini sauce and steamed string beans, it is advisable to eat the sesame noodles first. Oil-rich foods are usually concentrated protein foods.

- *Eat something raw with each snack-meal.* The enzymes in raw vegetables and raw fruit are an aid to digestion. Eating raw food with each meal reduces the work load for your enzyme-producing organs. It also frees the enzymes produced by your body to be used for repair work. The best digestive aids are raw, dark-green, leafy vegetables and raw apples.

- *Don't skip meals.* Your body needs a constant supply of carbohydrates for fuel. It also needs vitamins, minerals, enzymes, essential fatty acids, and protein for proper functioning and body repair. You would not expect your car to operate efficiently without the proper gas and oil. Why would you expect your body to function efficiently without a constant supply of the needed nutrients? It is advisable, however, to skip meals or eat significantly less if you do not feel well or if you are not digesting well. Give the body a chance to repair itself.

- *Don't overeat. Eat less than you think you need.* It takes 20 minutes for your body to realize it is satisfied. Stop eating *before* you are satisfied. Chances are, you will realize after 20 minutes that you have had enough to eat, unless you are experiencing a neurotic hunger. If you still feel hungry 30 minutes after you have finished eating, eat a little more of some *other* food. You will probably feel satisfied, unless you are experiencing a neurotic hunger. *Overeating makes you toxic, tired, overweight, less desirable, and sick.*

- *Chew all food to a baby-food texture. Don't inhale your food.* We are not vacuum cleaners. *Don't* count to 100 for each mouthful as some suggest. This can make you nervous, impatient, and drive you crazy. Relax, breathe, sit comfortably, and daydream when you chew. Just keep chewing

until the solids turn to a mushy *baby-food texture.* Nuts and seeds are not difficult to digest if you eat raw ones and if you chew them to a *baby-food texture.* Baby food is mush, regardless of the food's original texture. Your body cannot extract all the nutrients required for optimum health from insufficiently masticated food. Your health depends not only on the quality of the food you consume, but also on thorough mastication, which facilitates optimum assimilation.

- *Avoid eating when tired or stressed.* When stressed, people digest raw fruits more easily than all other foods. The addition of a few raw nuts or raw seeds (thoroughly chewed) does not usually complicate matters. If fatigue or stress is likely to continue for long periods, it is best to eat a snack but to eat less than usual. Digestion is closely linked with our emotional states. When upset, people either lose their appetite or become ravenous. Applied Kinesiology has shown the correlation between digestive functions and stress.

- *Food equals energy, not fatigue.* If you are in pain or feel sleepy, gassy, bloated or if you belch after a meal, consider the following as probable reasons:
  1) Inadequate mastication
  2) Overeating
  3) Eating too fast
  4) Eating too late
  5) Eating while stressed or fatigued
  6) Eating cooked or roasted fat-rich or oil-rich foods (animal foods, roasted seeds, or roasted nuts)
  7) Eating too large a portion of *raw*, oil-rich foods (seeds or nuts)
  8) Eating too many different kinds of foods at one meal
  9) Eating your meal randomly instead of one food at a time
  10) Gulping large quantities of fluids during or soon after a meal (small sips are fine)
  11) Food allergy

FOODS THAT FIGHT FOR OPTIMUM HEALTH, HUMAN RIGHTS, ANIMAL RIGHTS AND ECOLOGICAL EQUILIBRIUM

ORGANIC, WHOLE, UNREFINED GRAINS

Buying and Storage Hints

—Before purchasing, carefully inspect grains for insects.
—Avoid green grains; they are immature.
—Don't buy chipped or broken grains.
—Store grains in tightly sealed, dark jars away from light and heat.
—Use home-ground flour if possible. Grind grains just prior to use.
—Refrigerate leftover flour in dark, tightly sealed jars.
—If you buy flour, make sure it was shipped in refrigerated trucks and stored in the refrigerator in your health-food store.
—Use whole grains instead of cracked grains or flour; whole grains are nutritionally superior.
—Avoid buying toasted grains; additional nutrients are lost in toasting.

Variety

—Vary the grains in your diet.
—Prepare two cups of three different grains twice a week. This amount is sufficient for two people eating four or five snack-meals a day. The grains can be eaten at room temperature or slightly warmed. They also can be included in soups, wrapped in sheets of nori as vegetable sushi, blended with soy milk and eaten as a cream cereal, eaten whole like cereal with soy or other vegetarian milks, or combined with a variety of quick and tasty vegetable dishes.

—Try brown rice (short, medium, or long grain), wild rice, sweet rice, wehani rice, brown basmati rice, millet, buckwheat, corn, quinoa, amaranth, barley, oats, rye, wheat, and any other whole grains. Be adventurous.

COMMERCIALLY PREPARED WHOLE-GRAIN FOODS

General Advice

—Read labels for ingredients. "Sifted wheat" or "wheat flour" are refined wheat products. Avoid them.
—Eat salt-free and oil-free baked goods if possible. Occasional consumption of salt and oil will not harm you unless you have a particular intolerance.
—Select from all the commercially prepared foods listed below only if you are unable to use home-cooked whole grains. Commercially prepared whole-grain foods are useful as treats or when you are in a hurry.

Organic, Whole-Grain Breads

—Eat whole-grain sourdough breads made without the addition of yeast. Sourdough breads are predigested by the cultures and therefore are easier to digest.
—Eat breads containing no salt, oils, or sweeteners if possible.

Organic, Sprouted, Whole-Grain Breads

—Eat plain, sprouted, whole-grain breads instead of those containing nuts, seeds, and dried fruit. The nuts and seeds have been baked, thereby making them less nutritious and more difficult to digest. If you desire a richer, sweeter taste, eat some raw nuts or raw seeds and a piece or two of uncooked dried fruit with the sprouted grain bread.

Organic, Whole-Grain Flat Breads

—Eat corn tortillas and chapati without yeast, salt, oil, or sweeteners if possible.

Organic, Whole-Grain Crackers

—Do not use hydrogenated or partially hydrogenated oils or shortening. The crackers preferably should be free of salt, oil, yeast, or sweeteners.

Organic, Brown Rice Cakes

—Salt-free Lundberg rice cakes taste sweeter and have a more full-bodied flavor. Mochi Sweet rice cakes by Lundberg are sweeter tasting than any other rice cake on the market.

Organic, Whole-Grain Noodles

—Eat those that are salt-free if possible.
—Chew noodles to a *baby-food texture*. The tendency is to swallow unchewed bits and pieces. Improper mastication leads to indigestion and nutritional deficiencies.

ORGANIC FRESH VEGETABLES

General Advice

—Never buy limp or discolored vegetables.
—Refrigerate all vegetables to maintain optimum nutrient content.
—Wash all vegetables in warm or hot water with a natural vegetable cleanser. Because insecticides are oil-based, cold water with or without a cleanser will not remove the chemicals.
—Eat raw or lightly steamed vegetables. If you develop bloating and gas from eating raw salads, eat mostly steamed vegetables and gradually increase to larger salads over a period of months. Chew your salads to a *baby-food texture*. Insufficient mastication causes gas and bloating.

Dark-Green Vegetables

—Eat dark, leafy greens three times a day. They are your best source of vitamins, minerals (especially calcium), and chlorophyll. Romaine lettuce, watercress, spinach, parsley (it's not a decoration!), beet tops, collard greens, dandelion leaves, mustard greens, and turnip greens are the most popular. Broccoli, string beans, snow peas, zucchini, and Brussels sprouts are also excellent dark-green vegetables to consume frequently.

Organic Sprouts

—Consume sprouts daily. Try alfalfa, sunflower, daikon, mung, soybean, wheat berry, radish, buckwheat, or any other sprouts you enjoy.

Organic Yellow, Orange, White, and Light-Green Vegetables

—Eat three or four different colored vegetables daily for optimum nutrition. *Variety* on a daily and weekly basis is vital.
—Eat a variety of squash and root vegetables, especially in the late fall, winter, and early spring.

Sea Vegetables

—Eat seaweed twice a week. Seaweed supplies protein, vitamins (including some B_{12}), and minerals. It also helps to eliminate toxins from your body.
—Rinse and soak (to reduce salt consumption) hijiki, arame, kombu, and wakame, then simmer for 30 minutes.
—Eat nori raw or lightly toasted (hold over stove burner).
—Rinse dulse and eat it raw or cooked.

Organic, Unpasteurized (Raw) Sauerkraut

—Eat only *unpasteurized* sauerkraut because it supplies health-promoting bacteria and enzymes. Eat it daily, especially if you have digestive disturbances. Health-food stores sell unpasteurized sauerkraut made *without the addition of salt or vinegar* (Rejuvenative Foods, P.O. Box 8464, Santa Cruz, CA 95061, (408) 462-6715).

Fresh, Organic Vegetable Juices

—Because fresh vegetable juices are a highly concentrated food for the liver, dilute them with an equal part of water. Do not drink more than eight ounces of fresh diluted juice at one time.

—Swish or "chew" juices until saliva flows into your mouth thus enabling the digestive organs to secrete the proper amounts and types of digestive juices required for the particular juice you are drinking.

—*Don't gulp down your juices. Your body won't know what's coming down. It will be a shock and a strain on your digestive organs.*

—Consume juices immediately after squeezing to avoid the harmful effects of oxidation. (Don't wash the juicer or clean up the kitchen first!)

—Drink moderate amounts of fresh juices. Green juices are especially beneficial to your health. Do not defeat your good intentions by drinking too much juice or by drinking oxidized juices. Brown carrot juice is an example of an oxidized juice. Fresh carrot juice is bright orange.

—Use only *fresh*, diluted juices for fasting. If you decide to fast, read *several* books first. See the bibliography at the end of the book.

—Do not drink bottled juices if you want to achieve your optimum health. They are pasteurized, and their enzymes have been destroyed along with many vitamins.

ORGANIC FRUIT

Fresh, Organic Fruit

—Refrigerate all fresh fruit except bananas. Fresh fruit that has been left out at room temperature, for example, as a decorative center piece, is less nutritious.

—Don't buy or eat unripe fruit. Fruit ripened off the vine is never as nutritious or as tasty. The sugars in unripe fruit are not easily digested. (Ripe bananas are speckled brown.) Eat fruit that is in season.

—Wash fruit in *warm or hot* water with a vegetable and fruit cleansing liquid. Otherwise, you will not remove the oil-based insecticides. Wash organically grown fruit too because you can never be certain that it is free of insecticides unless you grow it yourself. The fruit could also be environmentally contaminated from nearby farms.

—Peel off the skin of nonorganic fruit. Washing the fruit never removes all the insecticides. Many nutrients are directly under the skin, so peel very thinly. Fruits are sprayed more than you can imagine. For example, most apples are sprayed as often as 15 times in one season. Unfortunately, insecticides do not just remain on the surface of the fruit; they penetrate into the fruit.

—Eat one to three pieces of fruit a day, depending on your tolerance for natural sugars.

—Eat citrus fruit (oranges, grapefruit, tangerines, etc.) twice a week. Too many will make your system too alkaline. (Citrus fruits are acidic, but they produce an alkaline reaction in the system.)

—Eat one apple a day. Eating an apple after a rich meal aids digestion.

Dried, Organic Fruit

—Do not eat dried fruits too frequently or in large quantities because the sugars in them are highly concentrated.

—Dried apricots taste much less sweet than other fruit.

—Expect to see dried fruit in varying shades of beige or brown. Dried fruits do not retain their original color. If apples are white, apricots bright orange, and pineapple yellow, you can be certain a preservative has been added.

—Soak dried fruit in water to soften it and bring out the flavor. Drink the soaking water or use it for cooking.
—Never eat more than *two* pieces of dried fruit at one time except for raisins or currants. (You should only consume one or two tablespoons of these.)
—Chew dried fruit to a liquid. The saliva will pour into your mouth as you chew and help to predigest the sugars.

Fresh, Organic Fruit Juices

—See advice previously given on fresh vegetable juices.

PLANT SOURCES OF CONCENTRATED PROTEIN

Organic Legumes

—Soak legumes overnight or sprout them for maximum digestibility. Beans, peas, lentils, peanuts, and any products made from these foods (e.g., tofu or tempeh) are legumes.
—Eat no more than one half a cup of legumes per day if you are also consuming other plant sources of protein; otherwise, maximum consumption should be one cup.
—Consume little or no plant sources of concentrated protein if you are trying to regain optimum health.

Organic Raw Nuts and Raw Seeds

—Eat only salt-free raw nuts and raw seeds.
—Refrigerate raw nuts and raw seeds, otherwise they will go rancid.
—Buy nuts and seeds in the shell for maximum freshness. When purchasing nuts without shells or seeds without shells, be sure they are not broken or too badly chipped.
—Buy nuts and seeds that were shipped in refrigerated trucks and kept refrigerated in your health-food store.

—Consume reasonable quantities of raw seeds, not more than two or three tablespoons a day.
—Consume reasonable quantities of raw nuts, not more than 10 or 15 at a time unless they are small nuts, in which case use a two or three tablespoon measure.
—Do not eat whole cashews without shells because they are almost always rancid. Eat raw cashew butter; it's less likely to be rancid. Rejuvenative Foods, P.O. Box 8464, Santa Cruz, CA 95061, (408) 462-6715.
—Consume only raw, unsalted nut or seed butters with no added oils.
—Eat pine nuts in the shell. They are usually rancid without shells.
—Consume sesame seeds raw to obtain maximum nutrition. Buy only mechanically hulled sesame seeds. Otherwise, chemicals have been used to remove their hulls.

THE SPICE OF LIFE

Organic Herbs

—Promote optimum health by using culinary herbs. Variety is important.
—Use fresh herbs whenever possible. Herb shops generally sell the freshest herbs. Buy them in small quantities to ensure maximum freshness.
—Avoid bottled, canned, or commercial herbs. *All culinary herbs have been irradiated unless the label specifically states "nonirradiated"!*
—Use large quantities of herbs to season your foods to reduce the desire for salt as a seasoning.
—Store herbs in dark containers away from light, heat, and moisture. The shelf life for most herbs is one year.

Seasonings

—Provided you are in good health and can tolerate the ingredients, use the following seasonings as needed: fresh lemon juice, organic apple cider vinegar, hato mugi vinegar, Tasty Gest, Dr. Bronner's Balanced Mineral Seasoning, Vegit, Lewis Labs Brewer's Yeast (unless you have Candida), salt-free mustard, Biosalt, low sodium tamari (not soy sauce), tekka, ume vinegar, Hot Stuff, miso (made with sea salt and *brown* rice), umeboshi plums, Sea Sauce (miso/ginger seasoning), mirin (a fermented sweetener), Quick Sip (something like tamari), *sweet* brown rice vinegar (Mitoku's has the best taste), toasted sesame oil (five or six drops per serving), and spicy sesame oil.

Organic Spices

—Use fresh spices whenever possible. Spices do not usually cause indigestion. See page 190 for most frequent causes of indigestion.
—Avoid black pepper because it is an irritant to the digestive tract. Cayenne, used in moderation, does not generally irritate the digestive tract.
—Squeeze garlic, onion, or ginger through a garlic press (the only garlic press that works is made by Zyliss), and use in fresh salad dressing or sauces. When heating sauces, add spices after the flame has been turned off to maintain maximum nutrient content.
—Use mild curry occasionally for variety.
—Grind cinnamon sticks or use whole.
—Grind or grate fresh whole nutmeg seeds.

ORGANIC OILS

—Bottles of oils do not grow on trees. Bottled oils are not a natural food. Your body cannot easily digest concentrated oils.
—Essential fatty acids are two of the most important nutrients to be found in oils. Highest concentrations are found in raw pumpkin seeds and raw walnuts.
—The best source of oils is obtained from raw whole foods such as raw nuts, raw seeds, and avocado.
—Because all animal foods are cooked, the essential fatty acids in them have been significantly destroyed.

—If you want to use an oil, use flaxseed oil. Choose a brand that is organic. The oil must be extracted without heat, light, oxygen, chemicals, or bleaching. Additionally it should contain no additives, preservatives, transfatty acids, or free radicals. The oil must be packed in opaque, black plastic bottles, otherwise light will enter and destroy the fatty acids. (Brown glass bottles do not block all light.) Both you and the health-food store *must keep the oil refrigerated* at all times to maintain its integrity. Respect the expiration date on the bottle.
—If you want to fry, only stir fry and then only in water. If you wish to add a small amount of oil, do so after the flame is turned off and just before you serve.
—If you use olive oil, use only the *extra* virgin olive oil sold in dark bottles.
—Refrigerate *all* oils.

ORGANIC SWEETENERS

—Avoid all sweetening agents, even honey, maple syrup, blackstrap molasses, barley malt, and mirin. If you are already experiencing optimum health, it is permissible to use these *occasionally*, which does not mean daily or every other day; it means on holidays, birthdays, and special occasions. If your health is less than optimum, it is best to obtain your sweetness from fresh fruit or slowly baked yams, sweet potatoes, baked Jerusalem artichokes, or squash. Interesting puddings and custards can be made with these foods.
—Avoid using fruit concentrates for sweetening. The sugars are far too concentrated to promote optimum health.
—If you want a sweeter taste, try substituting apple juice or white grape juice for liquids in recipes.
—Use Sucanat, an organic, totally unrefined cane sugar, as an excellent whole-food source of sweetness. It has more minerals than any of the above sugars, but it too should be used in moderation.

ORGANIC SALAD DRESSING

—Use fresh lemon juice or organic apple cider vinegar as the best liquid for most salad dressings. Vegetable stock or leftover steaming water can be added to extend the dressing.

—Add the following to the lemon juice and organic apple cider vinegar for variety: freshly squeezed garlic, ginger, or onion, (the best garlic press is made by Zyliss), fresh herbs, Quick Sip, quality oil, or a little raw seed or nut butter. Check the seasoning section for more ideas.

—Do not use oils with tahini or other seed or nut butters. They are foods already high in oil content.

WATER

—Drink six to eight glasses of water daily.

—Sip and swish every mouthful of water until you feel the saliva enter your mouth; then your body is ready to effectively utilize the water and its minerals.

—Drink 20 to 30 minutes *before* snack-meals or at least two to three hours *after* snacks, depending on the size of the snack. Drinking fluids (teas, juice, etc.) with or after meals dilutes digestive juices, interfering with digestion.

—If you must drink during or immediately after a meal, sip, sip, sip!

—Use glass water bottles instead of plastic. The plastic "bleeds" into the water. It is toxic and it tastes terrible.

—Mountain Valley and Evian are some of the reputable bottled waters. Mountain Valley water is a natural diuretic and thus very beneficial to your health because it helps your body to eliminate toxins.

—Drink water at room temperature. Icy cold water shocks your system.

NATURAL, NONTOXIC STIMULANTS

—Consume stimulants that are tonics (rejuvenative and healing to the body) as well as stimulants, like peppermint tea, Fo-TI, ginseng, Gotu-Kola. Coffee and tea are rarely grown organically. Even if naturally grown, regular consumption is not recommended. Some people can drink coffee or tea with no apparent side effects, but the majority of us aren't as fortunate. Remember, the side effects do not always show up immediately; some side effects are long term. One major concern is that caffeine is a strong diuretic and causes the loss of minerals, especially calcium.

SWEET TOOTH SATISFIERS

—Eat fresh fruit as the most healthful sweet tooth satisfier.

—For variety, slowly bake (250 degrees) naturally sweet foods such as fruits, yams, sweet potatoes, and squash. They provide a tasty change, particularly in the winter months when most fruits are out of season.

—Make use of the inexpensive and versatile apple. They can be baked whole (seasoned or unseasoned), sliced, diced, or grated. They can also be made into a delicious applesauce. You can create variety by adding one or more of the following: chopped raw nuts, freshly ground raw sunflower seeds, raw cashew cream (mix cashew butter with warm water), or freshly shredded coconut. Add these after cooking to keep the oils digestible. Oat flakes and spices, such as nutmeg and cinnamon, can be cooked with the apples to add zing.

—Keep freshly baked yams or sweet potatoes in the refrigerator. Nibble on them for an effortless, healthy, sweet treat. Yams or sweet potatoes may also be mashed, mixed with plain Edensoy milk (or other low-fat soy milk), seasoned with cinnamon and/or nutmeg, and baked as a custard or used as a pie filling.

—Make unsweetened jams at home when fresh fruits or berries are in season. Lightly cook the fruit in apple juice or white grape juice. Pectin or agar may be used as thickening agents. Preserved in mason jars, these delicately sweet jams can see you through winter. Avoid using fruit concentrates when making jams because the end product will be too sweet to be healthful.

—Try Lundberg mochi-sweetened rice cakes. They are sweeter tasting than ordinary rice cakes. Thoroughly chew rice cakes until they turn to a liquid. When chewed thoroughly, carbohydrates break down, with the help of saliva, into simple sugars. The resulting taste is quite sweet. Homemade jams; applesauce; and baked yams, sweet potatoes, or squash seasoned with cinnamon, nutmeg, raw nut, or seed butters can be spread on rice cakes for a delicious snack.

—*Every time you eat a sweet snack, be sure to have a hearty portion of dark greens after your snack.* The minerals in the dark greens help your body to metabolize the sugars. This is especially important if you have eaten a less healthy sweet.

—Chew your sweet treats even more thoroughly than other foods. Their high fat and high sugar content make them more difficult to digest.

4)SUPPLEMENTAL NUTRITION

Proper eating habits cannot always guarantee the optimum health you seek. You may have greater needs for certain nutrients because of a hereditary predisposition to a particular disease. Your job may expose you to toxins or external stresses (noise, bright lights, etc.) that increase your vitamin and mineral requirements. Flouridated water and air pollution also rob the body of essential vitamins and minerals. Finally, life's emotionally charged situations drain nutrients even further.

I recommend using foods or concentrated foods to obtain large amounts of specific nutrients. If you do not achieve the desired results within a reasonable time, supplements may be helpful. The science of nutrition is far from fully explored. No one knows the long-term results of taking megadoses of specific nutrients. Most foods are safe as long as you don't overeat.

The following chart provides information about the most common vitamins and minerals.

NUTRIENTS	BENEFITS: PART OF BODY/CONDITION	FOOD SOURCES
Vitamin A	Aging (premature), Alcoholism, Bones & Joints, Circulatory System/Heart, Diabetes, Ear Infections, *Energy, Eyes,* General Poor Health, Glands (thyroid), Hair, *Infections,* Intestines & Colon, Kidney (stones), Liver (hepatitis, jaundice, cirrhosis), Mouth (canker sores), *Mucous Membrane Protector,* Muscular System (dystrophy), Nervous System/Brain, *Pollution Protector,* Respiratory System (sinusitis), *Skin,* Stomach, *Stress* & related illnesses, Surgery (speeds recovery), Teeth & Gums, Urinary System (cystitis)	yellow & orange vegetables & fruit, dark green vegetables, sea vegetables (esp. *nori*), wheat grass, lemon grass, spirulina & other algae, liquid chlorophyll

NUTRIENTS	BENEFITS: PART OF BODY/CONDITION	FOOD SOURCES
Vitamin B Complex	*Aging (premature), Alcoholism,* Circulatory System/Heart, Digestive System (metabolism of carbohydrates), Diabetes, Ears, *Energy,* Eyes, General Poor Health, Glands (*adrenal exhaustion*), Hair, Infections, Intestines & Colon (improves peristalsis), Joints, Kidney (nephritis), Liver (hepatitis), Mouth (canker sores), Muscular System (cramps, weakness, muscular diseases, backache), Nails (growth), Nervous System/Brain, Reproductive System (premenstrual edema), Respiratory System, Skin, Stomach, *Stress,* Teeth & Gums, Urinary System (cystitis)	Lewis Labs Brewer's Yeast, whole grains, dark green vegetables, legumes, most raw nuts & raw seeds, blackstrap molasses (except B_1), root vegetables, B_{13}
Vitamin B_{12}	Alcoholism, Bones & Joints, Circulatory System/Heart (esp. *anemia & pernicious anemia*), Diabetes, General Poor Health, Glands (adrenal exhaustion), Intestines, Liver, Muscular System (diseases of the muscles), Nervous System/Brain, Respiratory System, Skin, Stomach, *Stress* & related illnesses	spirulina, fermented unpasteurized foods (tempeh, tofu, sauerkraut, etc.), sea vegetables, supplemental B_{12} (nasal, sublingual or injection)
Vitamin C	*Aging* (premature), *Alcoholism,* Bones & Joints, Circulatory System/Heart, Diabetes, *Drugs* (withdrawal), *Detoxifier,* Ears, Eyes, General Poor Health, Glands, Hair, *Infections,* Intestines & Colon, Liver, Mouth, Muscular System, Nervous System, Reproduction System, Respiratory System, *Stress* & related illnesses, Teeth & Gums, Urinary System	broccoli, sprouts (after exposure to sun), potatoes, cabbage, rose hips tea, citrus fruits, strawberries, cantaloupe, black currants, green bell peppers
Bioflavinoids (Vitamin P—Part of the Vitamin C-Complex)	Aging (premature), Anti-coagulant, Anti-oxidant, *Bruising,* Circulatory System/Heart (high blood pressure, *varicose veins* and other forms of capillary fragility), Diabetes, Eyes (retinal hemorrhages), Hemorrhoids, Joints (arthritis), Liver, Mouth (*bleeding*	citrus fruits (white of the peel is esp. rich), buckwheat, green peppers, grapes, apricots

NUTRIENTS	BENEFITS: PART OF BODY/CONDITION	FOOD SOURCES
	gums), *Radiation Sickness*, Reproductive System (miscarriages), Respiratory System, Skin, Synergistic to Vitamin C.	
Vitamin D	Aging (premature), *Aids Absorption of Calcium and Other Minerals*, Olcoholism, Bones & Joints, Circulatory System/Heart, Diabetes, *Energy & Vitality*, Eyes, Glands (thyroid), Intestines, Liver, Reproductive System (vaginitis), Respiratory System, Skin, Stomach (ulcers), Teeth & Gums	SUNLIGHT VITAMIN—This vitamin is formed on the skin. Do not shower for a few hours before or after exposure to the sun. Washing removes the oils that contain the precursors to Vitamin D. Sprouted seeds, raw sunflower seeds and mushrooms contain Vitamin D.
Vitamin E	*Aging* (premature), *Anti-oxidant*, Bones & Joints, Circulatory System/*Heart*, Diabetes, Ears, Eyes, Glands (thyroid & prostatitis), Hair, Intestines & Colon, Muscular System, *Reproductive & Sexual System*, Respiratory System, Skin (*sunburn*), Stomach, Urinary System, Varicose Veins	dark green vegetables, Brussels sprouts, whole grains, seeds (raw or sprouted)
Vitamin F Linoleic Acid Linolenic Acid	Circulatory System/*Heart*, Diabetes, Glands (adrenal), Intestines & Colon, Joints, Nervous System/Brain, Respiratory System, Skin (*external ulcers*), Teeth & Gums	raw pumpkin seeds, raw walnuts, raw sunflower seeds, raw almonds, avocados
Calcium	Alcoholism, *Bones* & Joints, Cataracts, Circulatory System/Heart, Diabetes, *Insomnia*, Intestines & Colon, *Muscular System* (cramps), *Nervous System*/Brain, Reproductive System (premenstrual tension & pain), Respiratory System, *Stress* & related illnesses, Teeth & Gums	dark green vegetables, sea vegetables (esp. arame, hijiki, wakame, kombu), spirulina, blackstrap molasses, whole grains, legumes, raw seeds, raw nuts (esp. raw almonds)
Chlorine	Digestion (increased hydrochloric acid production, vomiting), Hair (loss), Liver (detoxification aid, diarrhea)	sea vegetables, rye grain, watercress, avocado, cabbage, celery, cucumber, asparagus
Chromium	*Blood Sugar* Level Regulator (hypoglycemia, diabetes), Cholesterol Metabolism, Circulatory System/Heart	whole grains, Lewis Labs Brewer's Yeast, mushrooms

NUTRIENTS	BENEFITS: PART OF BODY/CONDITION	FOOD SOURCES
Cobalt	Pernicious Anemia (Cobalt is important for utilization of B_{12}!)	dark green vegetables, sea vegetables, most fruit
Copper	*Anemia*, Bones, Circulatory System/ Heart (edema), Hair (loss, color), Skin (bedsores), *Respiratory System* (impaired)	most raw nuts, raw seeds, legumes, dark green vegetables, raisins, whole grains, blackstrap molasses
Iodine	Circulatory System (esp. heart), Cretinism, General Poor Health, Joints (Arthritis), *Thyroid Disorders*	sea vegetables, swiss chard, turnip greens, watercress, peas, artichokes, garlic, pineapple, citrus fruit
Iron	Alcoholism, Circulatory System/Heart (*anemia*, blood), Diabetes, Intestines & Colon, Muscular System (improved performance), Nervous System (stress)/ Brain (memory), *Reproductive System & Sexual Organs (menstrual & pregnancy)*, Respiratory System, Teeth & Gums	dark green vegetables, sea vegetables (esp. arame, hijiki, nori) spirulina, Lewis Labs Brewer's Yeast, raw sunflower seeds, legumes, whole grains, dried fruit (prunes, raisins)
Magnesium	Alcoholism, Bones & Joints, Circulatory System/*Heart* (helps prevent cholesterol buildup), Diabetes, Digestive System (*natural antacid*), *Energy*, Intestines & Colon, *Muscular System* (cramps, spasms & twitches), Nervous System/Brain, *Stress* & related illnesses, Teeth, *Tranquilizer*, Wrinkles (eliminates premature)	dark green vegetables, raw nuts, whole grains, legumes, pineapple, blueberries, oranges, grapefruit
Phosphorous	Acid/Alkaline Balance, Alcoholism, Back Pain, Bones & Joints, Digestive System (carbohydrate metabolism), Circulatory System/Heart, Muscular System (cramps), Nervous System/ Brain, Sexual Organs (sexual drive diminished), *Stress* & Related Illnesses, Teeth & Gums, Weakness (general)	most vegetables (esp. potatoes), whole grains, most fruit, raw seeds & raw nuts, legumes
Potassium	Acid/Alkaline Balance, Alcoholism, Blood Pressure (lowers high blood pressure if due to excess salt), *Bones & Joints*, Circulatory System/*Heart*, Diabetes, Hypoglycemia, Intestines &	most vegetables (esp. steamed potatoes with peels), blackstrap molasses, whole grains, legumes, raw seeds, raw nuts, most fruits

NUTRIENTS	BENEFITS: PART OF BODY/CONDITION	FOOD SOURCES
	Colon, Respiratory System, Stomach (gastroenteritis), *Stress* & Related Illnesses, Teeth & Gums	
Selenium	*Aging* (premature; preserves tissue elasticity), Anti-cancer Properties, *Antioxidant*, Liver (cirrhosis), Mercury Poisoning, *Muscular System* (degeneration)	Lewis Labs Brewer's Yeast, sea vegetables, broccoli, whole grains, garlic, mushrooms, most vegetables
Sulfur	Anti-oxidant, Hair, Joints (arthritis), Nails, *Nature's Beauty Mineral*, Skin	cabbage, Brussels sprouts, radishes, turnips, onions, celery, string beans, watercress, kale, soybeans, raw nuts
Zinc	Alcoholism, Circulatory System/Heart, Diabetes, Eliminates Carbon Dioxide & Cadmium, Growth Process (bone formation, etc.), *healing* (speeds internal healing), Joints (arthritis), *Nails* (white spots on nails indicates deficiency), Nervous System/Brain, Night Blindness, *Reproductive & Sexual System* (prostatitis, infertility, sexual activity, maturity of sexual organs), *Skin* (healing of burns & wounds increases), Ulcers	*sprouted* pumpkin & sunflower seeds or sourdough breads, Lewis Labs Brewer's Yeast, mushrooms, onions, dark green vegetables

IMPORTANT: Chew all foods to a baby food texture for maximum assimilation. If you choose to take vitamin or mineral supplements, keep the pills in your mouth until saliva flows into your mouth. The flow of saliva signals that your body knows what's in your mouth. This technique will improve assimilation.

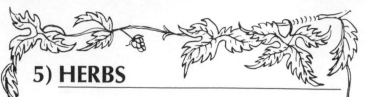

5) HERBS

Herbs have been used by doctors, medicine, women and men, witches and lay people since the beginning of time. Rich or poor, wise or uneducated, all alike have benefited from the healing qualities of herbs. Even the Bible states that herbs are to be our medicine. Today, in our age of modern medicine, many people are reverting to the use of herbs to cure or control disease, because herbs actually cure the cause of the disease, rather than merely masking the symptoms, and also because herbs, unlike drugs, rarely have any harmful side-effects.

Herbs act as catalysts within our body. As such, they help improve the body's own natural healing mechanism. Herbs can calm as well as stimulate. They can relieve pain, aid digestion, restore consciousness, raise or lower blood pressure, beautify the skin, rejuvenate internal organ functions, relieve spasms, act as an astringent, cure diarrhea or constipation, and heal wounds.

Store herbs in airtight, dark glass or tin containers away from the light, heat and dampness. Buy small quantities from shops that have a good turnover and keep herbs for only one year.

To make an infusion or herbal tea, use one-half to one ounce of the herb to one pint of water. Bring the water to a boil, then turn off the heat and pour boiling water over the herb. Cover and steep for ten minutes. Use only glass, enamel or porcelain pots. Drink the infusion, one mouthful at a time, throughout the day. Drink the tea cool or lukewarm, unless you wish to induce sweating, as in the case of a cold.

There are many books on the market that discuss herbs, their uses and methods of preparation. *The Herb Book* by John Lust and *Back to Eden* by Jethro Kloss are considered classics in the field.

Homoeopathic preparations stimulate the body's natural healing mechanism and, unlike herbal medicine, contain substances other than herbs. The doses of these preparations are minute highly stimulating. The strength is not, however, directly related to the herb in its crude form but rather to a dynamic power derived from that herb.

Consult a homoeopathic physician for the most efficient utilization of these herbal preparations.

ADRENALS—capsicum
ANEMIA—dandelion, comfrey
BLADDER—dandelion, chamomile, comfrey, uva ursi
CIRCULATION—capsicum, ginko
COLDS—comfrey, licorice, chamomile (drink or use as a vapor bath)
ENERGY—
♀ licorice, Fo-Ti, Dong Quai
♂ Gotu Kola, licorice, ginseng
EYESTRAIN—eyebright (drink and use as an eye wash)
GAS PAINS—catnip, thyme, ginger
GALL BLADDER—dandelion, yellow dock
HEART—sedative: mistletoe
    stimulant: wood betony, capsicum
KIDNEY—chamomile, dandelion, comfrey, uva ursi
HIGH BLOOD PRESSURE—capsicum, passion flower, garlic
IMMUNE SYSTEM—Taheebo or Pau D'arco Tea (not tea bags—inner bark only)
    Fresh garlic soaked 10 minutes in warm water (use garlic press), echinacea
INFECTIONS—golden seal, rose hips, echinacea
INSOMNIA—passion flower, german chamomile, valerian
LARGE INTESTINES—constipation: chickweed
    diarrhea: comfrey, peppermint, thyme
LIVER—dandelion, uva ursi, hops, alfalfa
LOW BLOOD PRESSURE—dandelion
LUNGS—comfrey, thyme, chickweed, fenugreek
MENOPAUSE—black cohosh, hops, Dong Quai
PANCREAS—dandelion, fenugreek
SEXUAL & REPRODUCTIVE ORGANS—
♀ ovaries: chamomile, Dong Quai
    general: red raspberry, Dong Quai
    ♂ prostate: ginseng
    urethra: ginseng
SORE THROAT—ginger (suck on a piece), golden seal
SINUS—golden seal, eyebright
STOMACH—comfrey, chamomile, fenugreek, ginger, lobelia
TENSION—mistletoe, passion flower, chamomile, valerian
TOOTHACHE—chamomile (hold in mouth around tooth)
TONIC—licorice, chamomile, dandelion, Gotu Kola, ginko, ginseng

6)MEDITATION

Meditation is a very beneficial practice for all people. It can give you clarity of thought, free you from excessive tensions, improve physiological as well as psychological health and yield a more fulfilling spiritual awareness. Meditation is particularly healthful to high-strung, very active individuals who need a time once or twice a day to stop and get in touch with themselves and everything around them. Although such individuals may find it difficult to stop racing and unwind enough to meditate, it is possible with repeated practice. The rewards will prove great enough to merit the initial effort. It appears that the more a person needs meditation, the more difficult it is to find the time to achieve this state of mind.

If meditation seems to you too inextricably tied up with gurus and devotees, don't be discouraged. It is possible to learn the skill from such people and then take it home for your own personal use. On occasion you may need to return to your teacher in order to refresh your skill, but you can remain aloof from the traditional and ritualistic aspects of these institutions if you so desire.

There are many different types of meditation. I am not about to say that one is better than the next. Whichever works for you is the best for you. Transcendental Meditation is one of the more common and easily located schools of meditation. Because many articles have been written on the benefits of Transcendental Meditation in prestigious scientific journals, it is perhaps the best-known to the general public. This does not mean, however, that is the best form of meditation. Other types of meditation, like those, for example, that do not use a mantra but instead focus on a shape or color, can achieve good results if they are practiced correctly. The key is to give your all to the technique of your choice. Be patient and you will be rewarded.

Meditation and massage go hand in hand. The relaxed state of awareness achieved through meditation can be called upon when receiving a massage and can enhance its benefits. Furthermore, a person who practices meditation regularly will come to the massage therapist with less tension. The therapist will thus be able to reach deeper into the essence of the subject, instead of having to work with all the tensions that accumulate from week to week. In other words, greater and deeper releases will be achieved to provide more fulfillment and rewards for both the therapist and the receiver.

7)GENERAL AIDS

There are many general health aids that can be purchased from both health food stores and department stores. These devices can be used in your home to improve your general health. Some are inexpensive and others are quite the opposite, but they are all worthwhile investments. This section describes some of the more common and popular of these devices and briefly discusses the benefits from the use of each.

SLANT BOARD

Slant boards can be purchased from sporting goods stores. They can also be made inexpensively. Cover a plank with some sort of padding, tack it down, and voila: you have a slant board. The board should be a little longer than you are tall and at least as wide as is your body with your arms by your side. Place the slant board at a 20-45° angle, then lie on it with your feet up and your head down. Rest in this position once or twice a day for fifteen to twenty minutes. The regular use of a slant board will improve your general circulation, relieve eyestrain and fatigue, improve hearing and vision, help sinus conditions, encourage new hair-growth, benefit your complexion, relieve the almost constant downward pull of gravity on your internal organs, improve the circulation in your legs and feet, and better your overall health. To relieve lower back strain, place a bolster cushion or two bed pillows under your knees and rest your head on a folded towel or small pillow that is approximately 1 1/2-2 inches thick.

FOOTSIE ROLLER

Footsie rollers can be purchased in your local health food store. With the purchase comes a brochure explaining how to use it. Regular use of your roller will improve the circulation to your legs and feet, as well as the flexibility of your knee joints. It will also improve your overall health, because the roller stimulates all the reflex points on the bottom of your feet which correspond to all your internal organs and all parts of your body. Use the footsie roller while reading, relaxing or watching television.

KENKOH SANDALS

These sandals have tiny, raised projections on the top surface of the sole of the shoe which constantly make contact with the sole of your foot. Walking with these sandals constantly stimulates all the reflex points on the soles of your feet, improves your overall circulation, and relieves tired, cold or aching feet. Wear the sandals only briefly at first, in order to allow your feet time to adjust to the constant stimulation.

TRAMPOLINE

Trampolining is fast becoming a very popular form of exercise. It's fun, and it really does do wonders to improve your overall health. Trampolining also burns more calories than most other types of exercise. So, if weight's your problem, this is the solution you've been looking for. Do not purchase one of the cheapest models, as it will not endure as much wear-and-tear as one better made. When beginning your exercise routine on the trampoline, position the trampoline near a wall so that you can use the wall for balance. Don't overdo it at first. Begin with one or two minutes at a time, then gradually increase the length of time you spend rebounding. The first time most people get on a rebounder, they are so excited that they jog and jump for five or ten minutes. The next day they regret it because their legs ache. It's not advisable to strain your muscles. Restrain your enthusiasm at the outset, and gradually lengthen the time you spend on your trampoline.

IONIZER

If you live in or near a large city, it is impossible to breathe clean air. Even country dwellers are now experiencing the results of polluted atmospheres. Your lungs, skin and liver could use a break. A top-quality ionizer will greatly improve the quality of the air you breathe. Two to four per room is ideal. Ionizers also improve your concentration and give you more energy.

HUMIDIFIER

The winter months leave your house much too dry for healthful living. A humidifier replaces the moisture needed to keep your skin young and healthy-looking. It also helps to improve your overall health. Purchase a top quality unit, otherwise you are wasting your money.

PLANTS

Fill your apartment or house with plants. They consume your carbon dioxide and produce fresh oxygen for you to breathe. Apart from this life-giving quality, they are beautiful to behold and sensitive, responsive friends to have in your home.

INVERSION BOOTS

Inversion boots are sold in sporting goods stores. You clip the boots onto your ankles and hook the boots onto a chin-up bar. Then you hang upside down. You can also do sit-ups or kneebends while hanging. Even if you do nothing but hang, you will improve your circulation, relieve eyestrain, encourage hair-growth, relieve sinus congestion, release low back pain and improve your complexion. Your general health will also improve. Be sure the chin-up bar is secure. Raise and lower yourself slowly, and you'll have no problems.

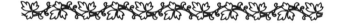

How To Locate A Holistically Oriented Doctor

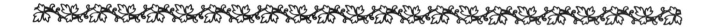

Everything is going well in your life. You are healthy and happy. Suddenly you or someone you love is stricken with a serious illness. You would like to treat the illness by natural methods rather than with conventional drug therapy, but you don't have a family doctor, let alone a doctor that is holistically oriented. How does one go about locating a holistic doctor? They aren't yet listed in the yellow pages under "Holistic M.D.'s." The easiest way I know is to ask friends, or else visit or call your local health food store and ask for a few recommendations. Holistically oriented doctors always send supplements they have prescribed. The employees and the owners get feedback from the doctor's patients, and after a few years of feedback, you can be sure the local health food store knows who is achieving results and who isn't. Call various doctors. Speak to them or their assistants in order to determine which doctor would be right for you. Then, make an appointment. It would be advisable, of course, to locate a physician before you get sick and to have a general check-up. Then, if you should need medical attention, you will be assured the services of a doctor who is already familiar with you and your body.

Unless you can find a nutritionally oriented internist who also uses homoeopathic herbs as a method of treatment, I strongly recommend that you consult two doctors. Generally speaking, nutritionally oriented doctors do not use herbs in their practice and homoeopathic doctors do not always stress nutritional therapy. Most doctors specialize in either nutrition or homoeopathy, as

the study of both would require many years of education and training. Therefore, combine the best of two fields of medicine to attain the best health care you possibly can. The nutritionally oriented internist will treat your malady with dietary and nutritional therapy, while the homoeopathic doctor will treat your condition with herbal remedies. Homoeopathic doctors have all studied orthodox medicine before specializing in homoeopathy. The Queen of England has her own private homoeopathic doctor, and the Royal Family has had a homoeopathic doctor in their service for four generations. For those of you who have no knowledge of homoeopathic medicine or who have been made skeptical of it by orthodox physicians, you might feel more confident with a homoeopathic doctor knowing that the Queen of England thinks it's good enough for her and her family.

Finally, you can top off this dynamic approach to your health with visits once a month, or more often if recommended, to a chiropractor. A chiropractor will realign your body and thereby make it easier for your body to heal itself. If your body is capable of healing itself, these three medical practitioners will, in combination, help it happen.

As a final reminder, don't forget to add massage and self-massage to your repertoire of healing aids. Massage will help to cleanse the body and mind so as to make the healing process more certain. Locate the best massage therapists, as well as the best homoeopathic doctors and chiropractors, by getting recommendations from your local health food store.

Where to Locate Health Services

Throughout *The Magic of Massage* many references have been made to institutions, specialty physicians and various products in an attempt to provide you with the best possible aids for the betterment of your emotional and physical health. Although many more such services and products are available, they are not included simply for lack of space. I have attempted to cover the fundamentals necessary for peak health, but no doubt you will discover on your own many other valid and useful systems and accessories that will add to your growing health. The following pages catalogue in alphabetical order the aids, accessories and institutions discussed in this book. A list of services, or partial list in some cases, accompanies most recommendations. I have also added personal commentary in those instances where personal experience deems it appropriate.

ACUPUNCTURE

American Association of Acupuncture and Oriental Medicine
50 Maple Place
Manhasset, New York 11030
(516) 627–0309
Services: Referral to qualified acupuncturists in every area of the United States, all of whom are registered in a computerized directory.

ALEXANDER LESSONS

American Center for the Alexander Technique, Inc.
129 West 67th St.
New York, New York 10023
(212) 799–0468
Services: Lessons, training, lectures

CHIROPRACTORS

International College of Applied Kinesiology
P.O. Box 25276
Shawnee Mission, Kansas 66225
(913) 268–8771
Services: (I.C.A.K. is not a college. It is an educational organization that teaches those who are licensed to diagnose. Send a stamped, self-addressed business envelope for addresses of wholistic practitioners in your vicinity.

FOOTSIE ROLLER

Matrix International
21 Dry Dock Ave.
Boston, Massachusetts 02210
Services: Manufacturer of footsie rollers and other health aids. Most health food stores carry footsie rollers, but if you are unable to obtain one in your area, try writing to the above address.

HOMOEOPATHY

National Center for Homoeopathy
1500 Massachusetts Ave. N.W., Suite 41
Washington, DC 20005
Services: Directory of U.S. Homoeopathic Physicians available for a small fee.
Dr. T.C. Cherian
141 Sound Beach Avenue
Old Greenwich, Connecticut 06870
(203) 637–8632

The author has had many years of experience with Dr. Cherian and his innovative approach to homoeopathy. She recommends him highly because he has consistently achieved excellent results with her many referrals. If you live in New York, Connecticut or New Jersey, take advantage of Dr. Cherian's expertise.

INVERSION BOOTS

Gravity Guidance, Inc.
1540 Flower Ave.
Duarte, CA. 91010
Services: Mail-order inversion boots, Gravity Guider and Dr. Robert Martin's book *The Gravity Guiding System*

IONIZER

Bionaire Corp.
565A Commerce St.
Franklin Lakes N.J. 07417
Services: Top quality ionizers/air purifiers

MUSIC

Halpern Sounds
Back Roads
200 Tamal Vista Boulevard #409
Corte Madera, California 94925
1–800–845–4848
Services: Mail-order tapes and records of music appropriate for massaging, meditating or listening

NUTRITIONALLY ORIENTED PHYSICIANS

American Board of Nutrition
9650 Rockville Pike
Bethesda, Maryland
Write to this organization and they will send you the addresses of physicians in your vicinity who are certified by the American Board of Nutrition. *NO PHONE CALLS.* You must send a stamped, self-addressed business envelope or you will get no response.

REBOUNDERS-TRAMPOLINES

Most sporting goods stores and some health food stores now sell this very efficient piece of exercise equipment. A hint! Don't buy the cheap models because they won't hold up under constant daily use.

REFLEXOLOGY

National Institute of Reflexology
P.O. Box 12642
St. Petersburg, Florida 33733
Services: Instruction, certification, referrals, the sale of books

ROLFING

Rolf Institute
P.O. Box 1868
Boulder, Colorado 80306
(303) 449–5903
Services: Training, certification, referrals

SHIATSU

Ohashi Institute
A Nonprofit Educational Institution
12 West 27th St., 9th Floor
New York, New York 10001
(212) 684–4190
Services: Basic, intermediate and advanced classes, birth educator workshops as well as a variety of other workshops. Free Open House Wednesday Evenings 8:30–10:00 P.M.

SILVA MIND CONTROL

Silva Mind Control
25 East 20th St.
New York, New York 10003
(212) 477–4400
Services: A wonderful course! Learn to reprogram your mind to improve yourself and the world.

SWEDISH MASSAGE

Swedish Institute, Inc.
875 Avenue of the Americas
New York, New York 10001
(212) 695–3964
Services: Instruction, certification, preparation for licensing, massage practitioner references, graduate courses.
The Swedish Institute is the oldest massage school in the U.S.A. and the only massage school that is accredited by the U.S. Department of Education.

TOUCH FOR HEALTH

Touch for Health Foundation
1174 North Lake Avenue
Pasadena, California 91104–9975
(818) 794–1181
Services: Basic classes, instructor-training workshops, professional programs, basic & advanced education referrals to certified independent instructors and to professionals who use TFH techniques.

THEnterprises
1200 North Lake Avenue
Pasadena, California 91104
(818) 798–7893
(800) 826–0364
Services: Sale of books, charts and other related health products

TRANSCENDENTAL MEDITATION

I recommend this type of meditation because it works. Every major city in the U.S.A. has a center or a qualified teacher listed in the white pages under Transcendental Meditation Program.

BIBLIOGRAPHY

(Addresses are given for those books available only by mail.)

ACUPUNCTURE

ACUPUNCTURE
Felix Mann, M.B.
Vintage Books, Random House, Inc.

AN OUTLINE OF CHINESE ACUPUNCTURE
The Academy of Traditional Chinese Medicine
Chan's Corporation
P.O. Box 478
Monterey Park, California 91754

ANIMAL ISSUES

DR. PITCAIRN'S COMPLETE GUIDE TO
NATURAL HEALTH FOR DOGS & CATS
Richard H. Pitcairn, D.V.M., Ph.D., & Susan
Hubble Pitcairn
Rodale Press, Inc.
33 East Minor Street
Emmaus, Pennsylvania 18049

COOKBOOKS

THE COOKBOOK FOR PEOPLE WHO LOVE
ANIMALS
P.O. Box 1418
Umatilla, Florida 32784

EAT FOR STRENGTH: A VEGETARIAN
COOKBOOK
Oil Free, Sugar-Free, Dairy-Free
Agatha Thrash, M.D.
Thrash Publications
Route 1, Box 273
Seale, Alabama 36875

THE McDOUGALL HEALTH SUPPORTING
COOKBOOK
Vol. 1 and Vol. 2
Mary A. McDougall
New Century Publishers, Inc.
220 New Brunswick Road
Piscataway, New Jersey 08854

NO OIL, NO FAT VEGETARIAN COOKBOOK
Trudie Hoffman
Professional Press Publishing Co.
13115 Hunza Hill Terrace
Valley Center, California 92082
(619) 749-1134/749-1135

THE VEGAN KITCHEN
Freya Dinshah
The American Vegan Society
501 Old Harding Highway
Malaga, New Jersey 08328

DIET & NUTRITION

DIET FOR A NEW AMERICA
John Robbins
Stillpoint Publishing
Box 640
Meeting House Road
Walpole, New Hampshire 03608
1-800-847-4041

DIET FOR A SMALL PLANET (10th Edition)
Frances Moore Lappe
(Important: The 10th edition is totally revised
and offers the latest advice on vegetarianism;
the older editions are outdated.)
Ballantine Books

FASTING CAN SAVE YOUR LIFE
Herbert M. Shelton
Natural Hygiene Press
A Division of The American Natural Hygiene
Society
1920 W. Irving Park Road
Chicago, Illinois 60613

FASTING: THE ULTIMATE DIET
Allan Cott, M.D.
Bantam Books

THE MIRACLE OF FASTING
Paul C. Gragg, N.D., Ph.D.
Health Science
Box 7
Santa Barbara, California 93103

HOW TO GET WELL
Paavo Airola, Ph.D., N.D.
Health Plus Publications
P.O. Box 22001
Phoenix, Arizona 85028

McDOUGALL MEDICINE
John A. McDougall, M.D.
New Century Publishers, Inc.
220 New Brunswick Road
Piscataway, New Jersey 08854

THE McDOUGALL PLAN
John A. McDougall, M.D. & Mary A.
McDougall
New Century Publishers, Inc.
220 New Brunswick Road
Piscataway, New Jersey 08854

NUTRITION ALMANAC
Nutrition Search, Inc.
John D. Kirschmann
McGraw-Hill Book Co.

PREGNANCY, CHILDREN & THE VEGAN DIET
Michael Klapper, M.D.
P.O. Box 959
Felton, California 95018-0959

VEGAN NUTRITION: PURE AND SIMPLE
Michael Klapper, M.D.
P.O. Box 959
Felton, California 95018-0959

HERBS

BACK TO EDEN
Jethro Kloss
A Life Line Book
Woodbridge Press Publishing Co.
P.O. Box 6189
Santa Barbara, California 93111

THE HERB BOOK
John Lust
Bantam Books

HOMEOPATHY

DR. SCHUESSLER'S BIOCHEMISTRY (THE
TWELVE BIOCHEMIC REMEDIES)
J. B. Chapman, M.D.
New Era Laboratories, Ltd.
39 Wales Farm Road
London, England W36XH

HOMEOPATHIC MEDICINE
Harris L. Coulter, Ph.D.
Formur, Inc.
St. Louis, Missouri

MASSAGE & RELATED TOPICS

ARE YOU TENSE?
THE BENJAMIN SYSTEM OF MUSCULAR
THERAPY
Ben E. Benjamin
Pantheon Books

DO-IT-YOURSELF SHIATSU
Wataru Ohashi
E.P. Dutton

HEALING MASSAGE TECHNIQUES: A STUDY
OF EASTERN AND WESTERN METHODS
Frances M. Tappan
Reston Publishing Company, Inc.
A Prentice-Hall Company
Reston, Virginia 22090

LOVING HANDS
Frederick Leboyer
Alfred A. Knopf, Inc.

THE MASSAGE BOOK
George Downing
Bookworks Book
Random House

MASSAGE, MANIPULATION AND TRACTION
Sidney Licht, M.D.
Robert E. Krieger Publishing Co., Inc.
Melbourne, Florida 32901

TOUCH FOR HEALTH
John F. Thie, D.C. with Mary Marks, D.C.
DeVorss & Company, Publishers
1046 Princeton Drive
Marina del Rey, California 90291

THE USE OF MASSAGE IN FACILITATING
HOLISTIC HEALTH
Robert Henley Woody, Ph.D., Sc.D.
Charles C. Thomas, Publisher
Bannerstone House
301-327 East Lawrence Avenue
Springfield, Illinois 62717

ZEN SHIATSU
Shizuto Masunaga with Wataru Ohashi
Japan Publications, Inc.
200 Clearbrook Road
Elmsford, New York 10523
1174 Howard Street
San Francisco, California 94103
P.O. Box 5030 Tokyo International
Tokyo 101-31, Japan

Index